COLORFUL PICTURE BOOK OF PSALMS

"Taste and see that the LORD is good; blessed is the one who takes refuge in him."

Psalm 34:8

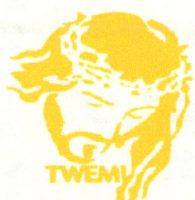

Copyright © 2020 The Word Evangelical Ministries Inc.
www.amazon.com/author/tweminc
All Rights Reserved.

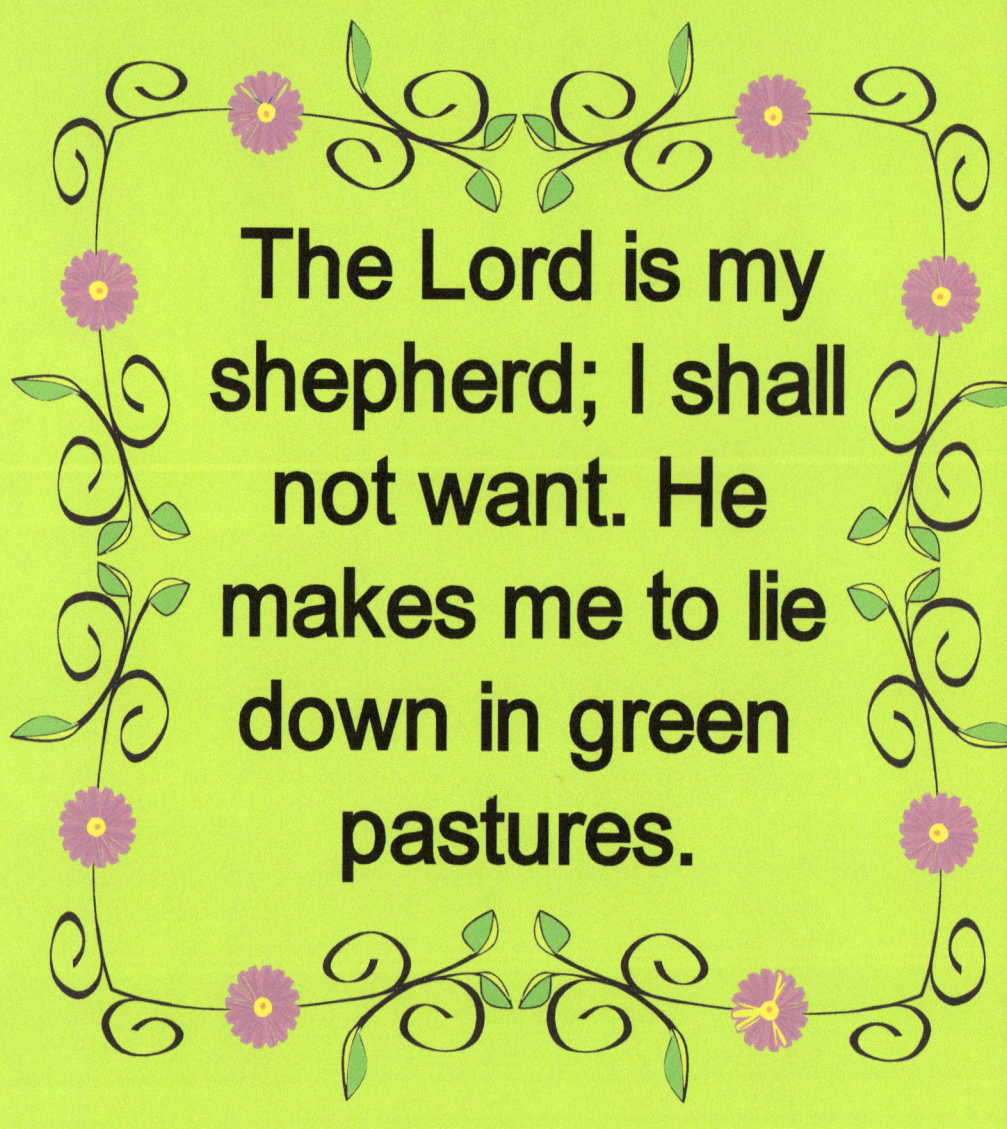

The Lord is my shepherd; I shall not want. He makes me to lie down in green pastures.

Psalm 23:1-2

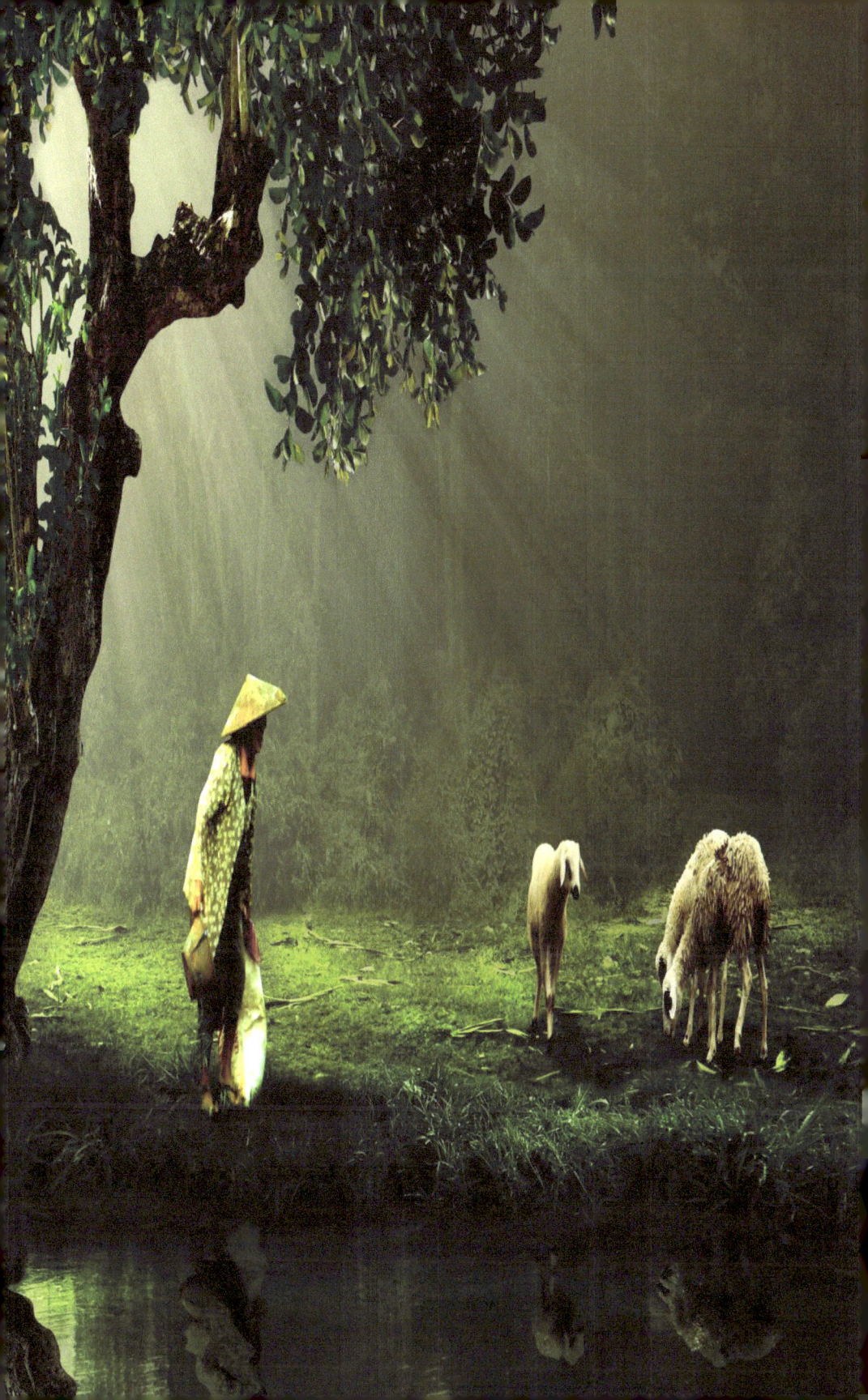

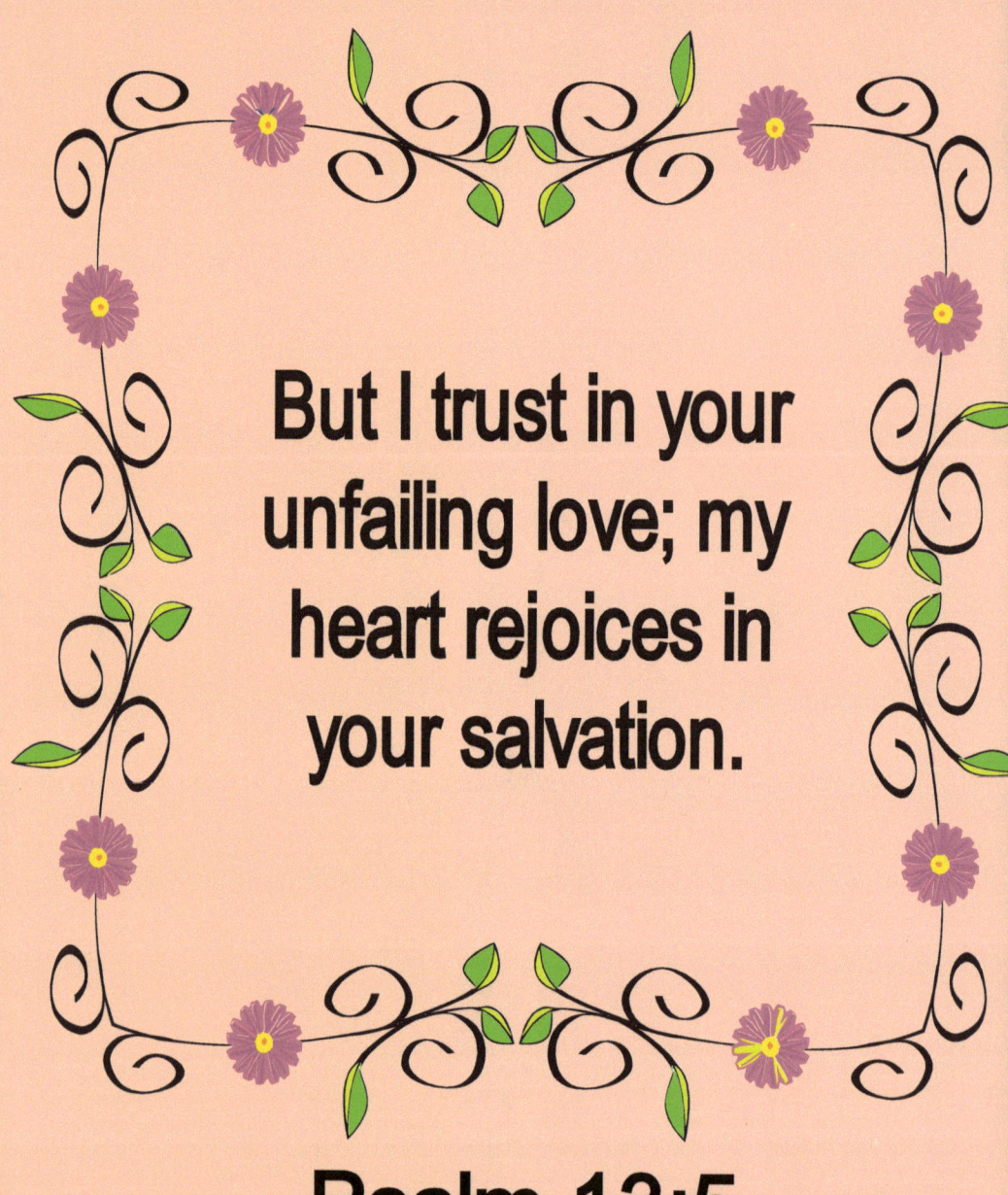

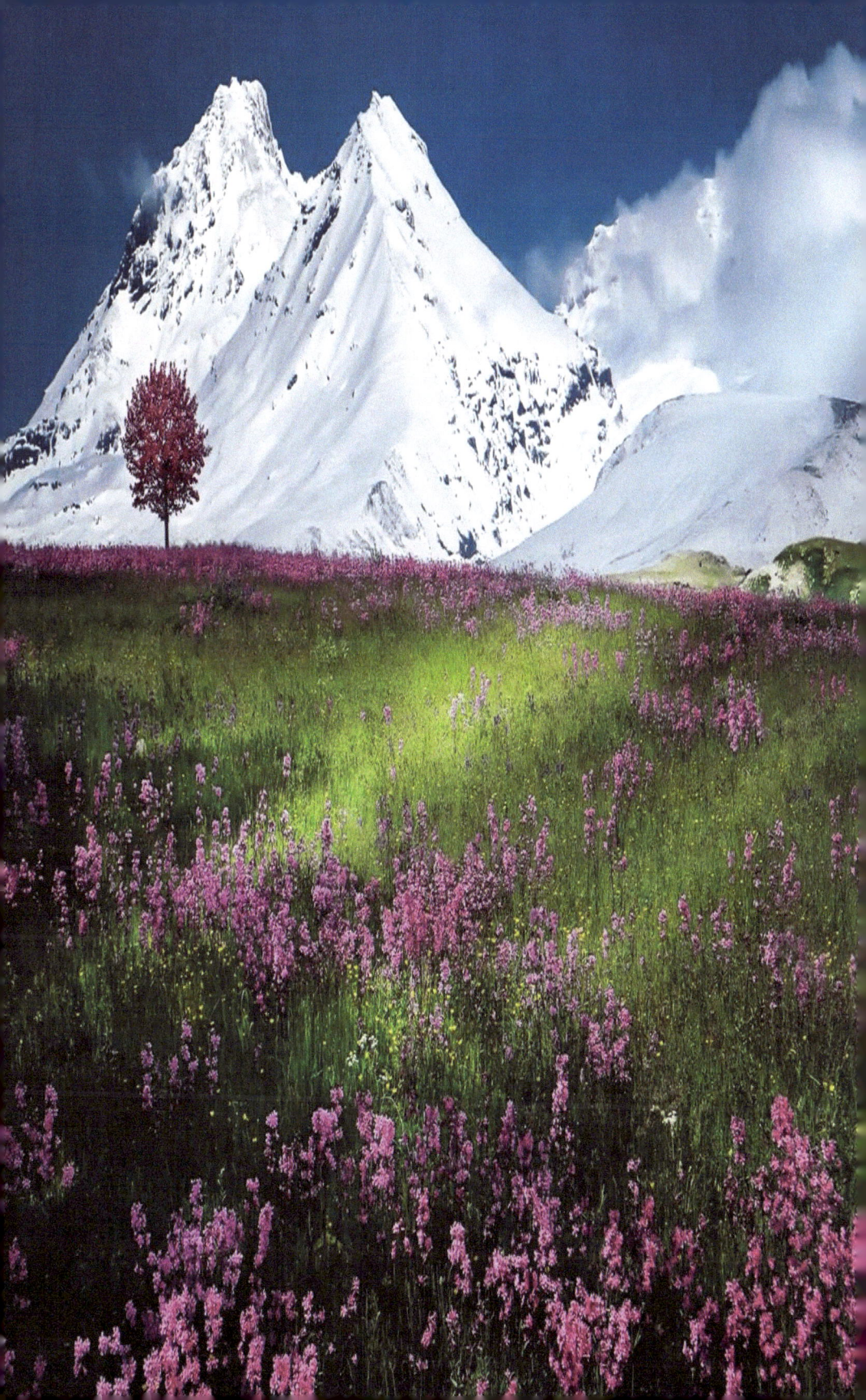

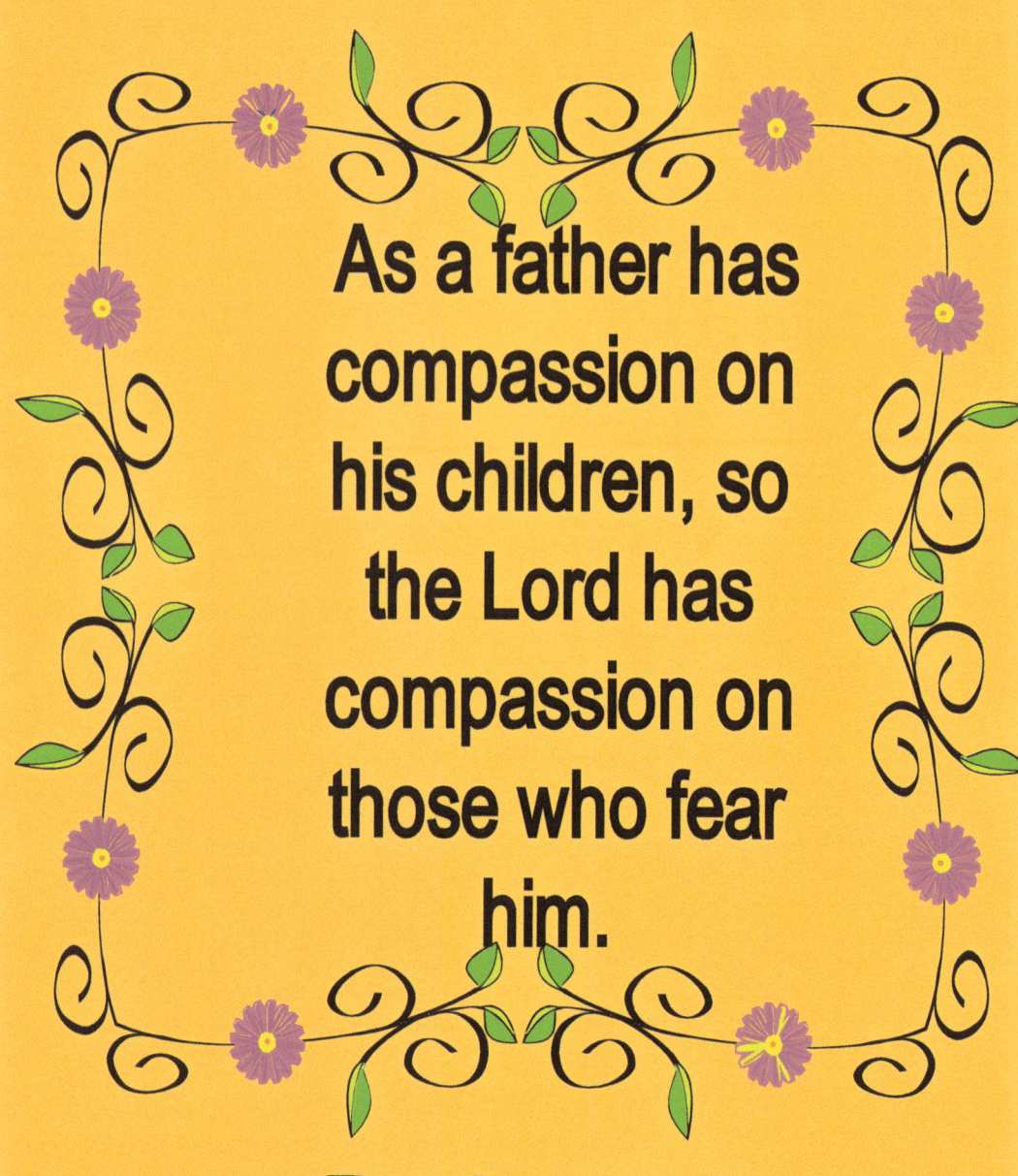

As a father has compassion on his children, so the Lord has compassion on those who fear him.

Psalm 86:5

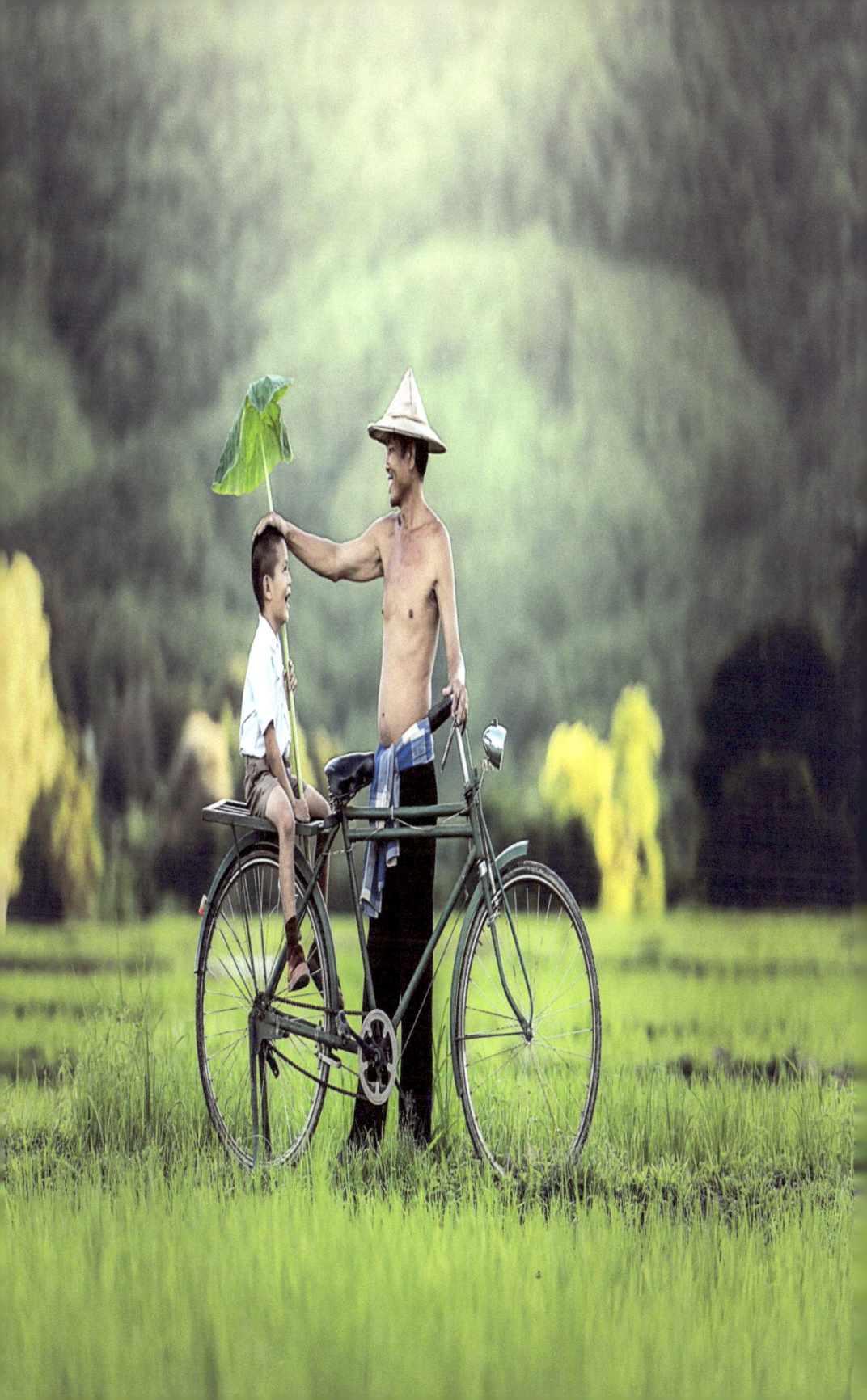

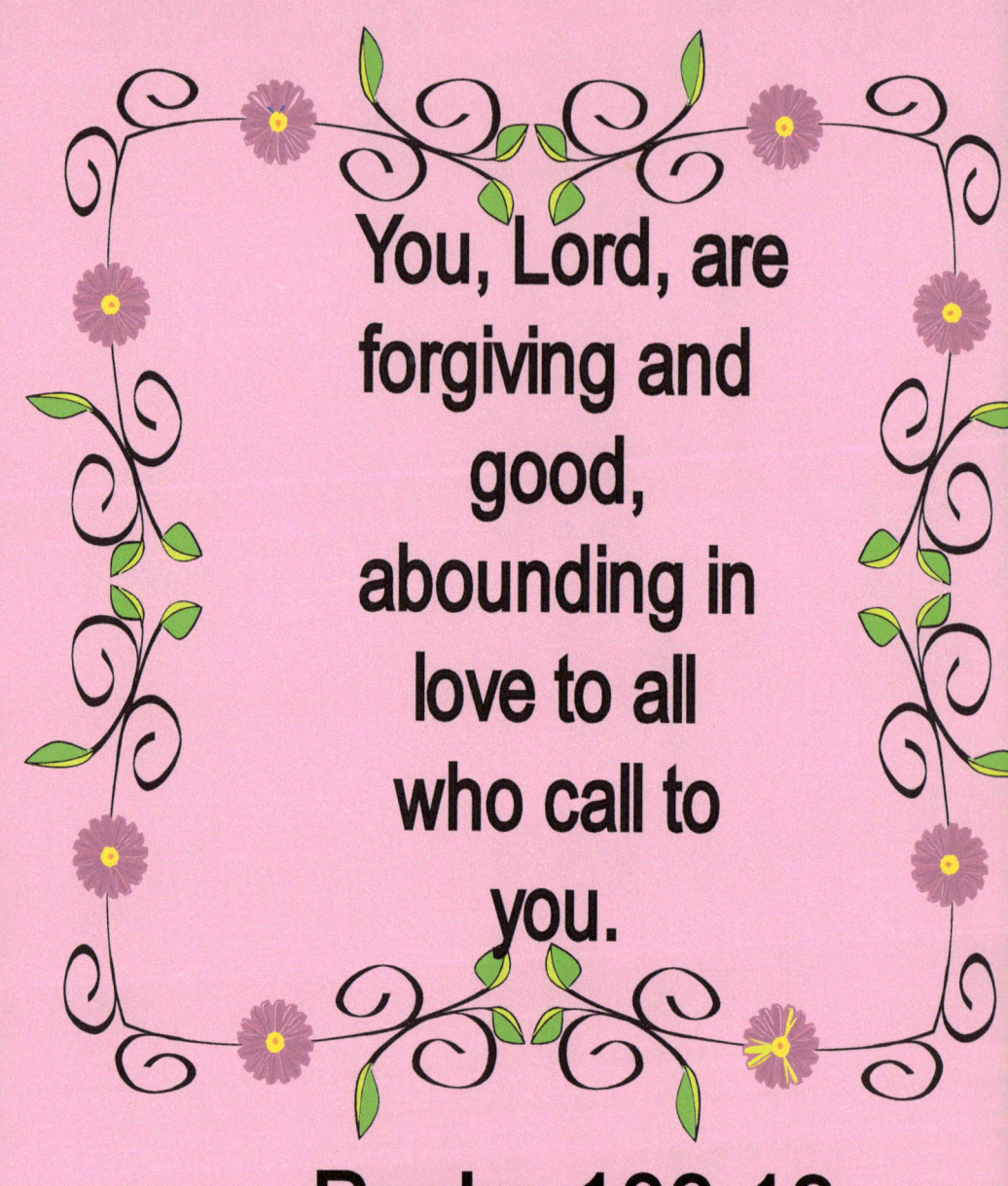

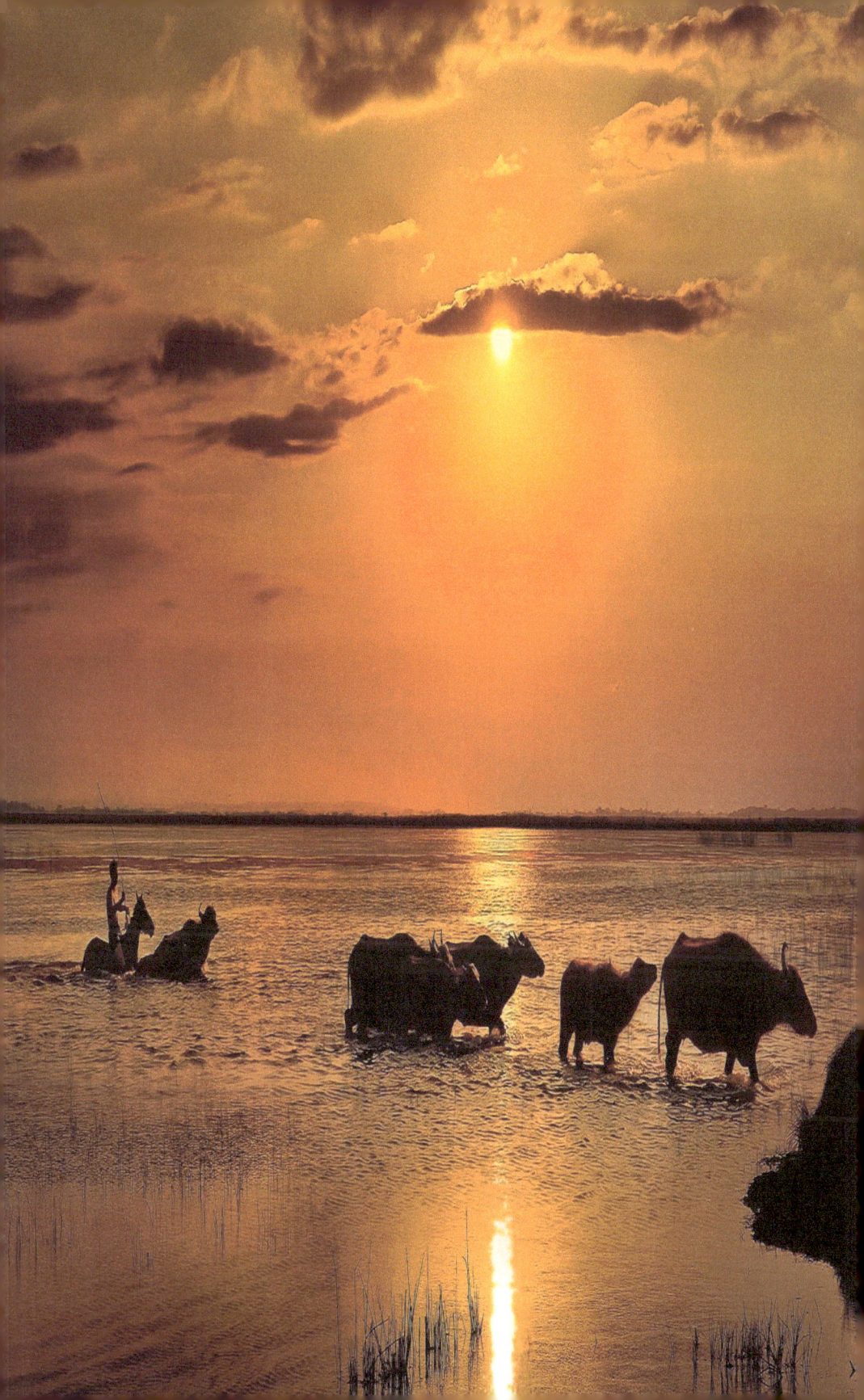

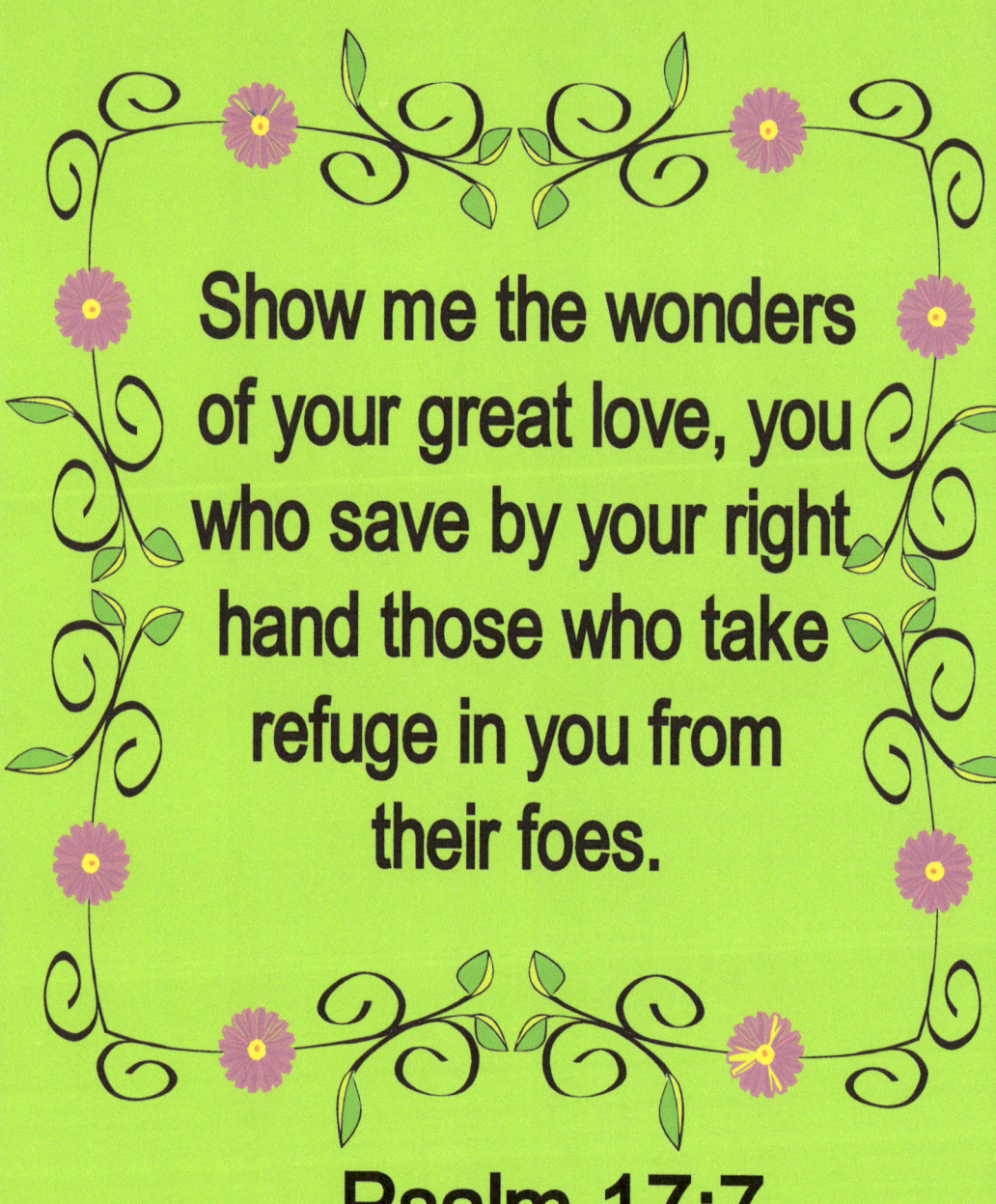

Show me the wonders of your great love, you who save by your right hand those who take refuge in you from their foes.

Psalm 17:7

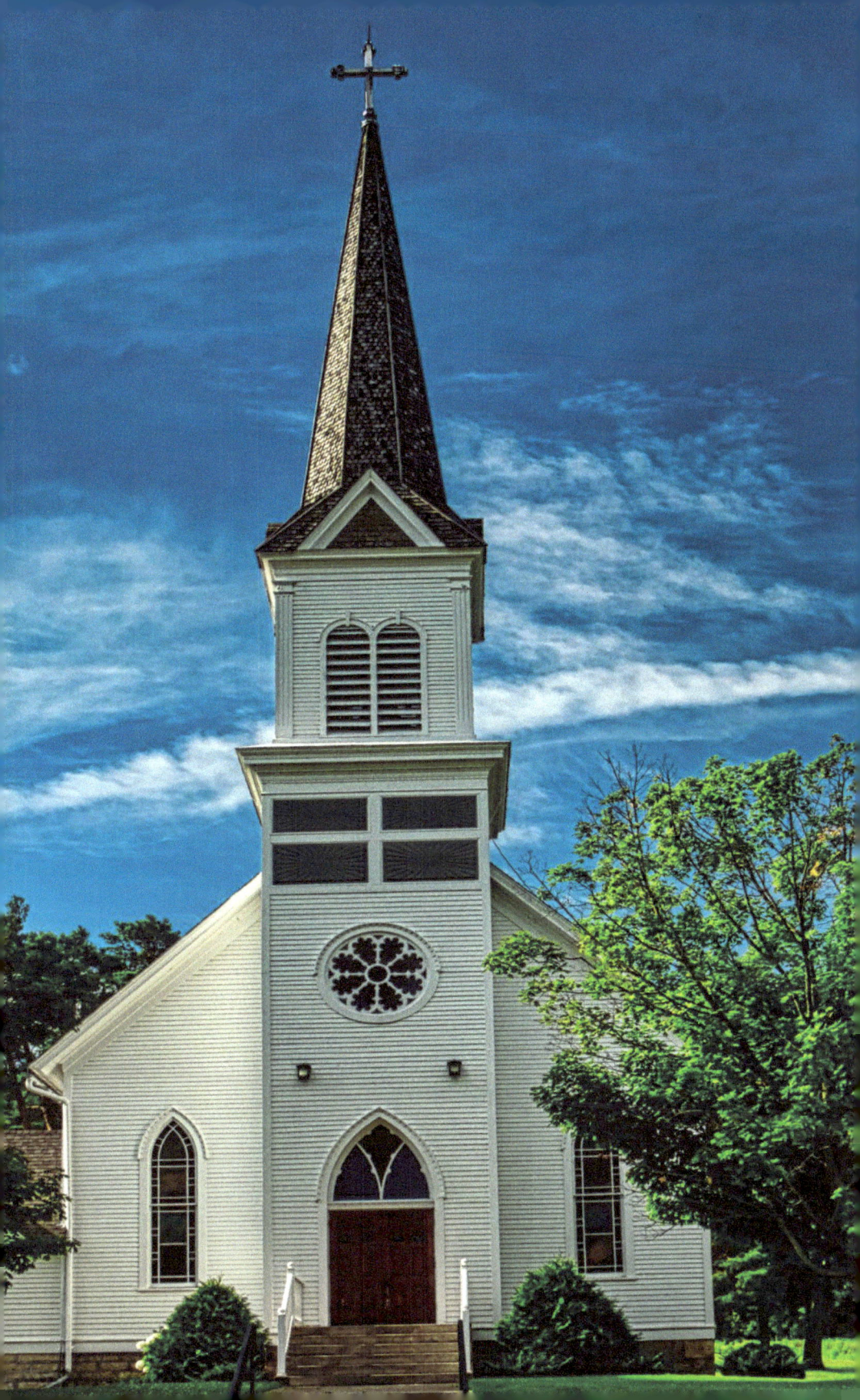

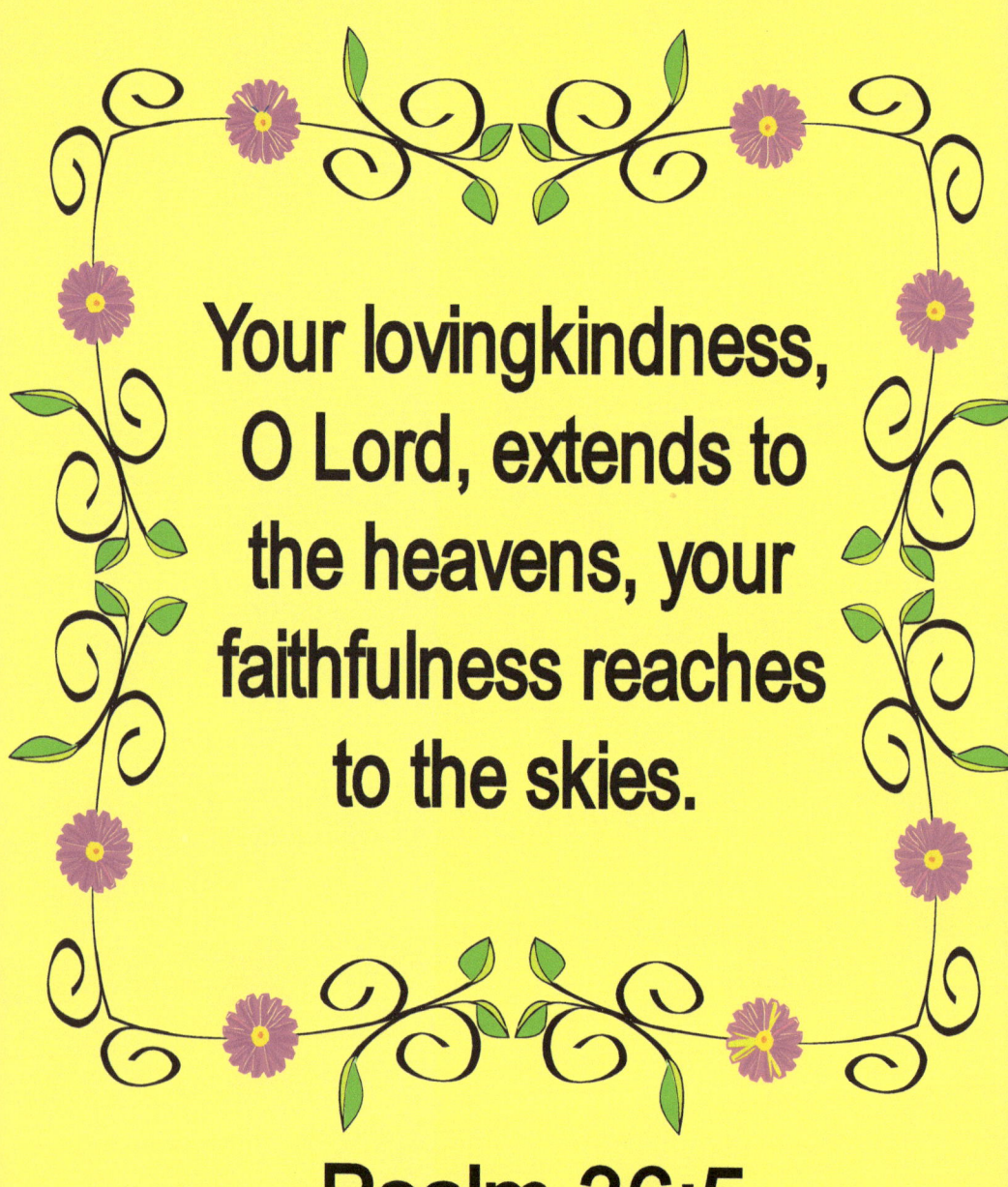

Your lovingkindness, O Lord, extends to the heavens, your faithfulness reaches to the skies.

Psalm 36:5

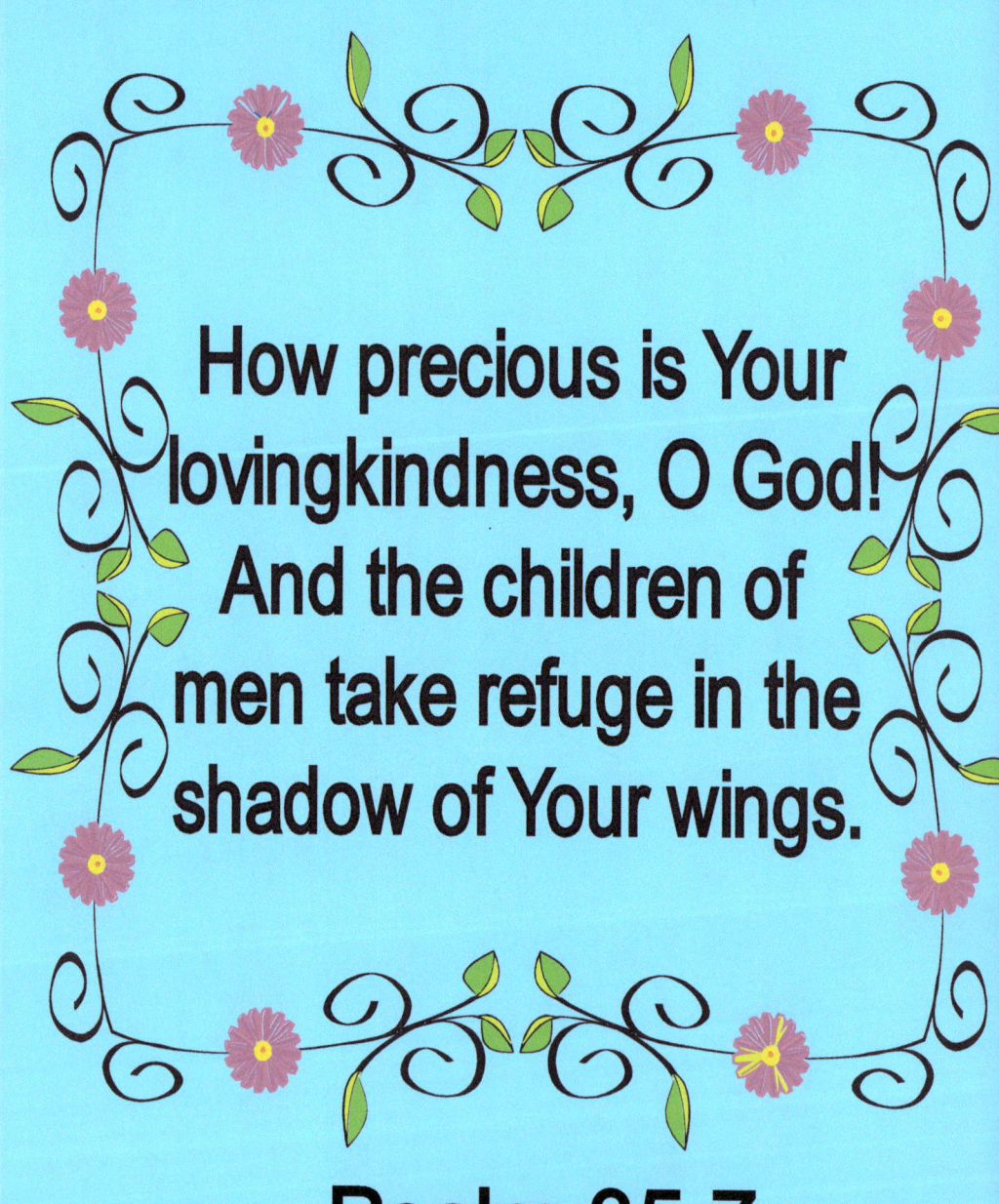

How precious is Your lovingkindness, O God! And the children of men take refuge in the shadow of Your wings.

Psalm 35:7

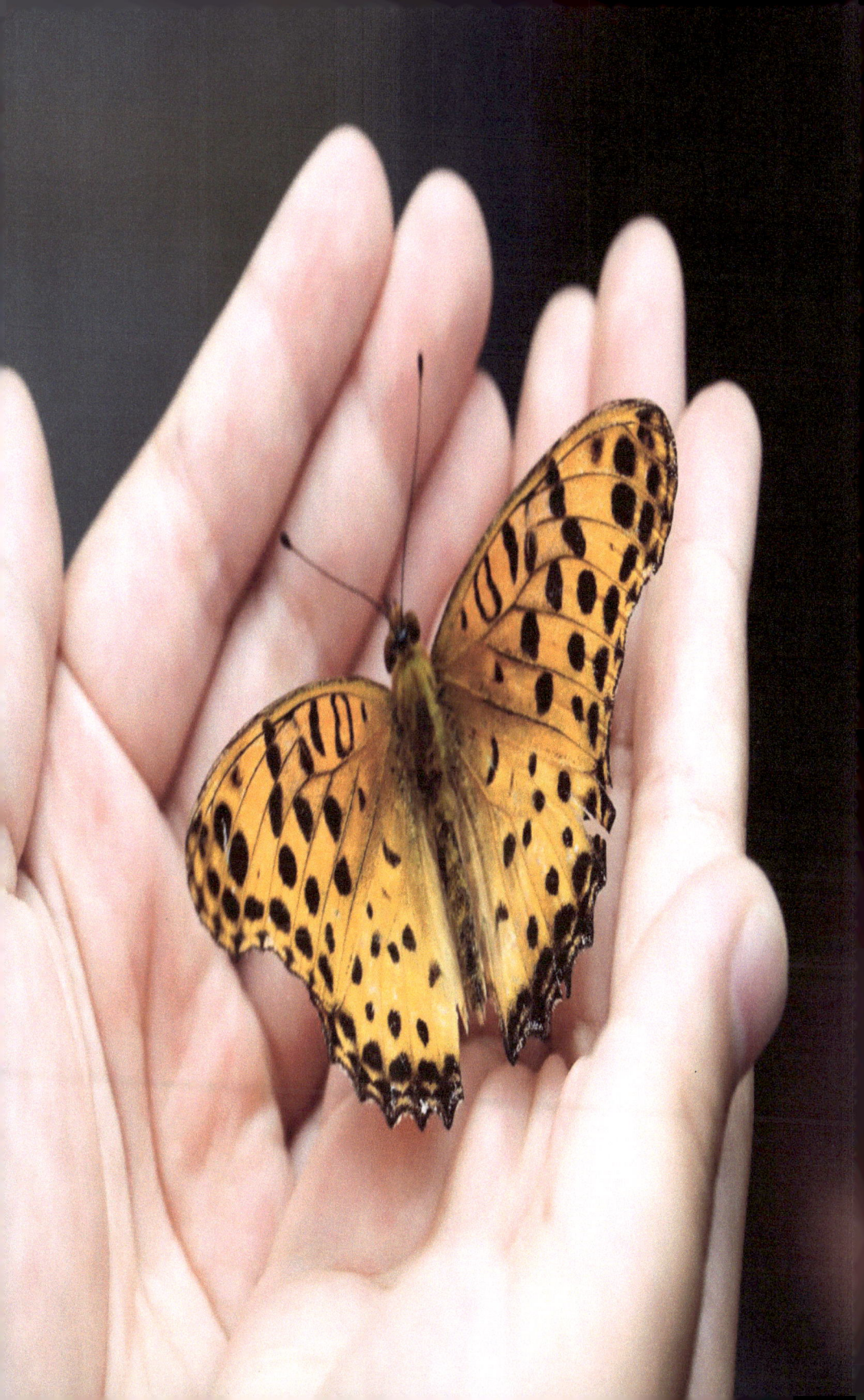

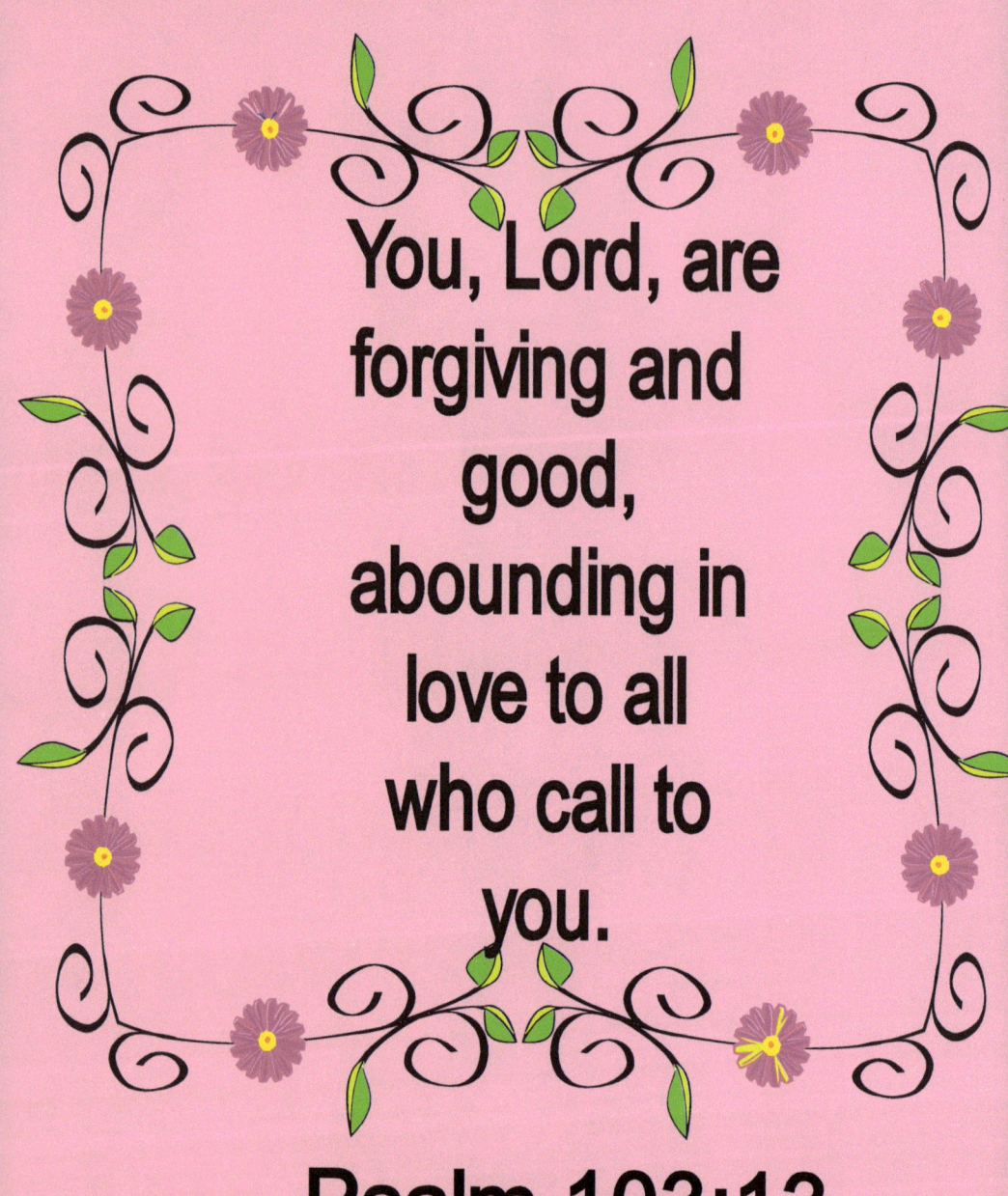

You, Lord, are forgiving and good, abounding in love to all who call to you.

Psalm 103:13

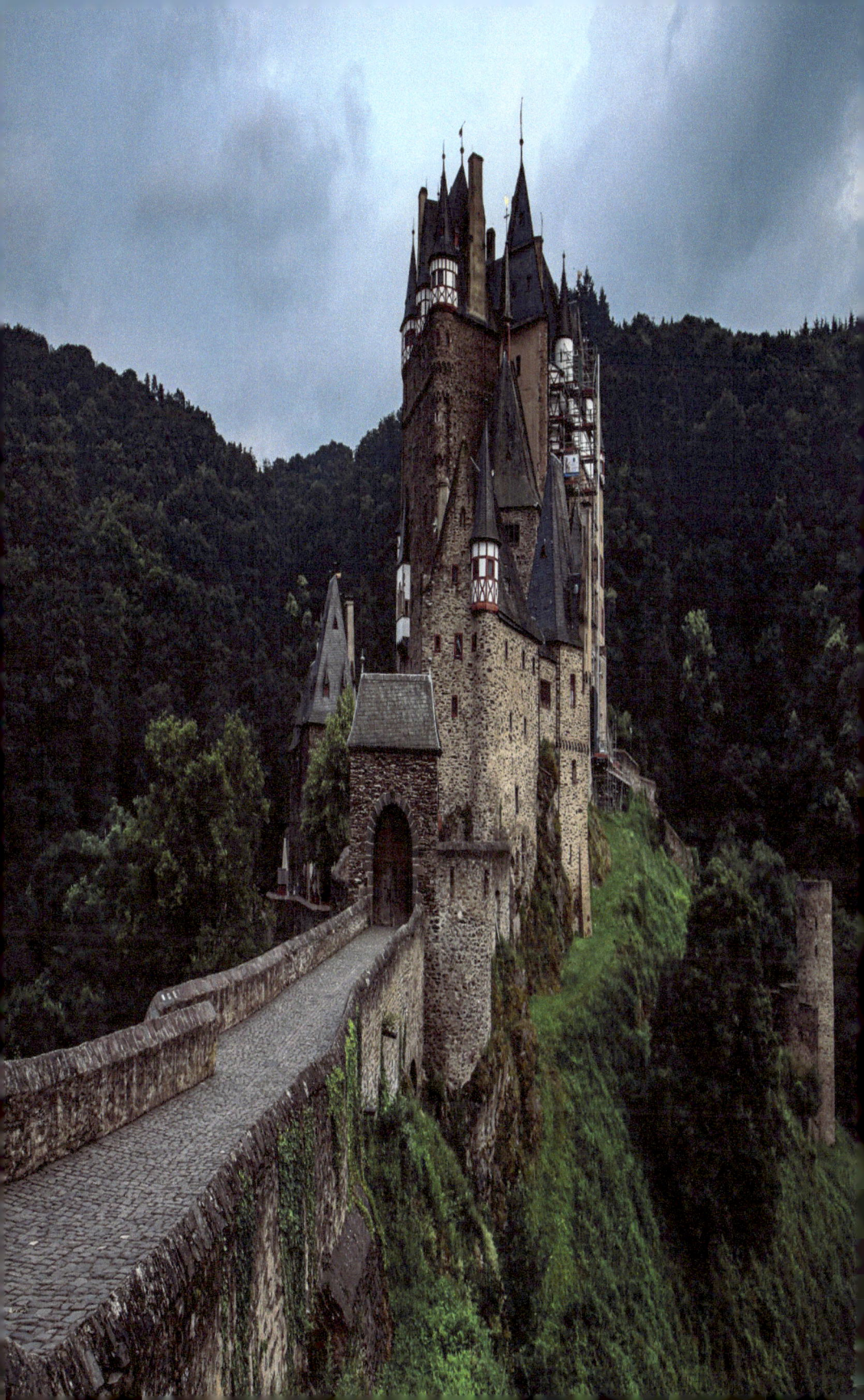

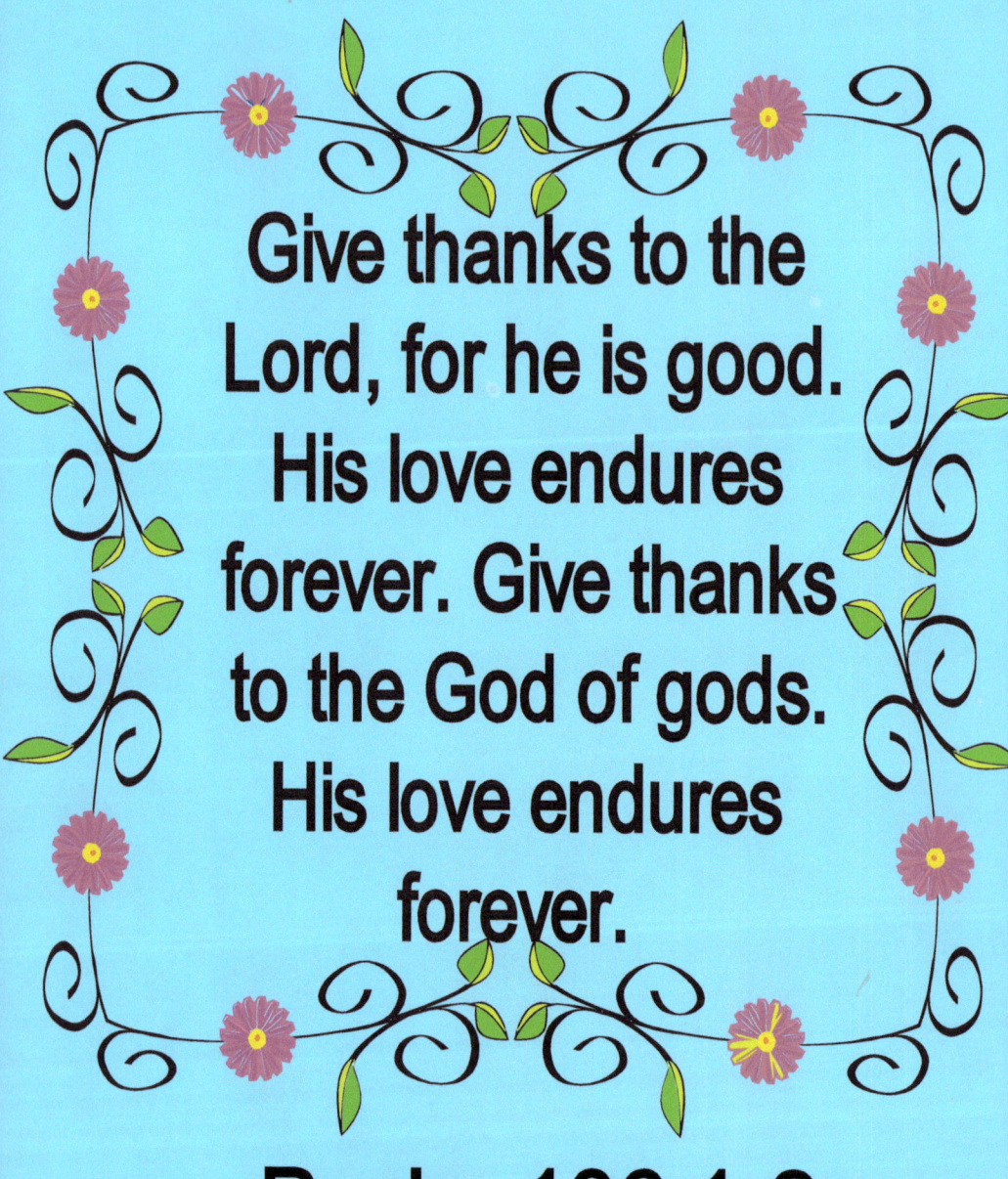

Give thanks to the Lord, for he is good. His love endures forever. Give thanks to the God of gods. His love endures forever.

Psalm 136:1-2

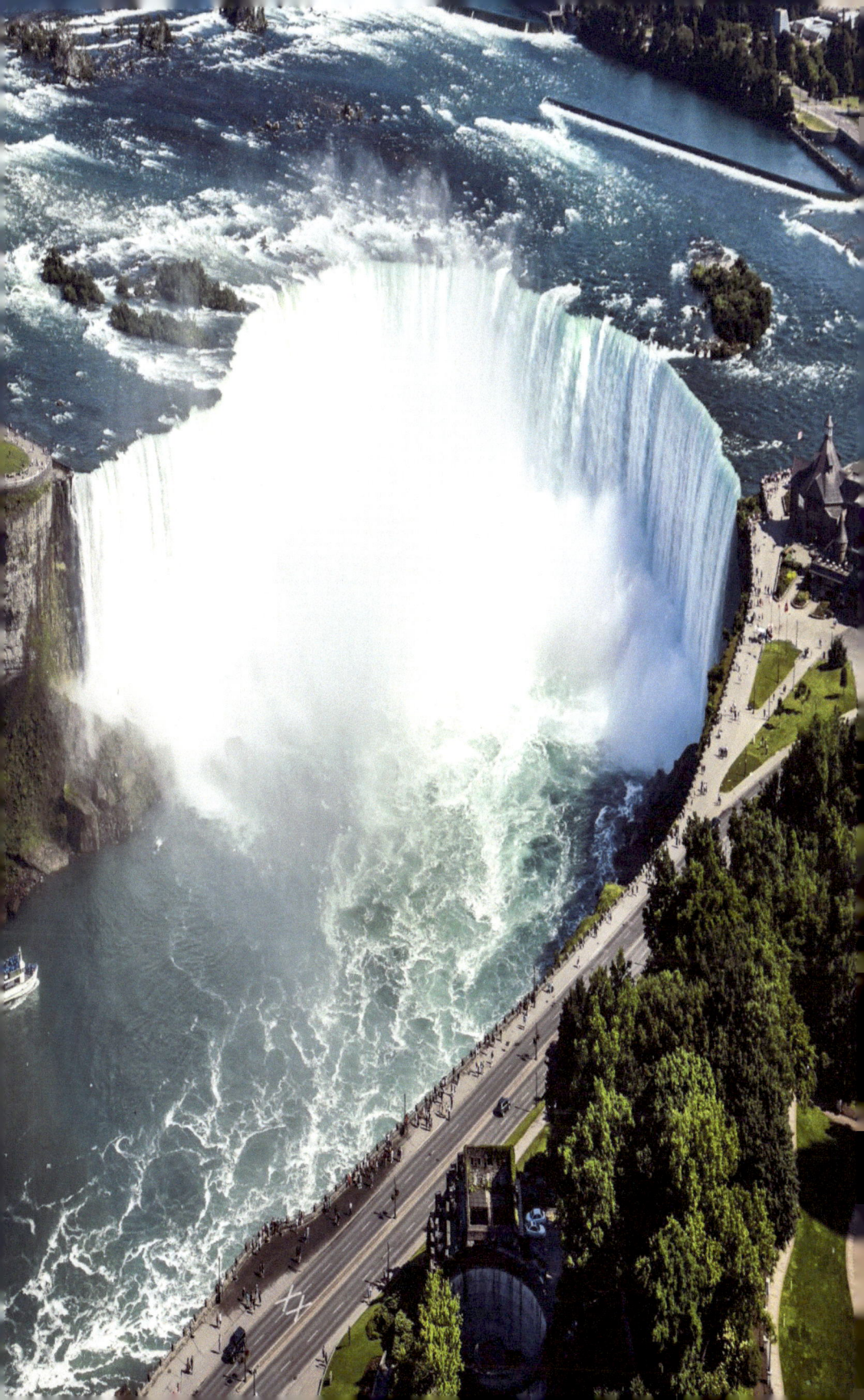

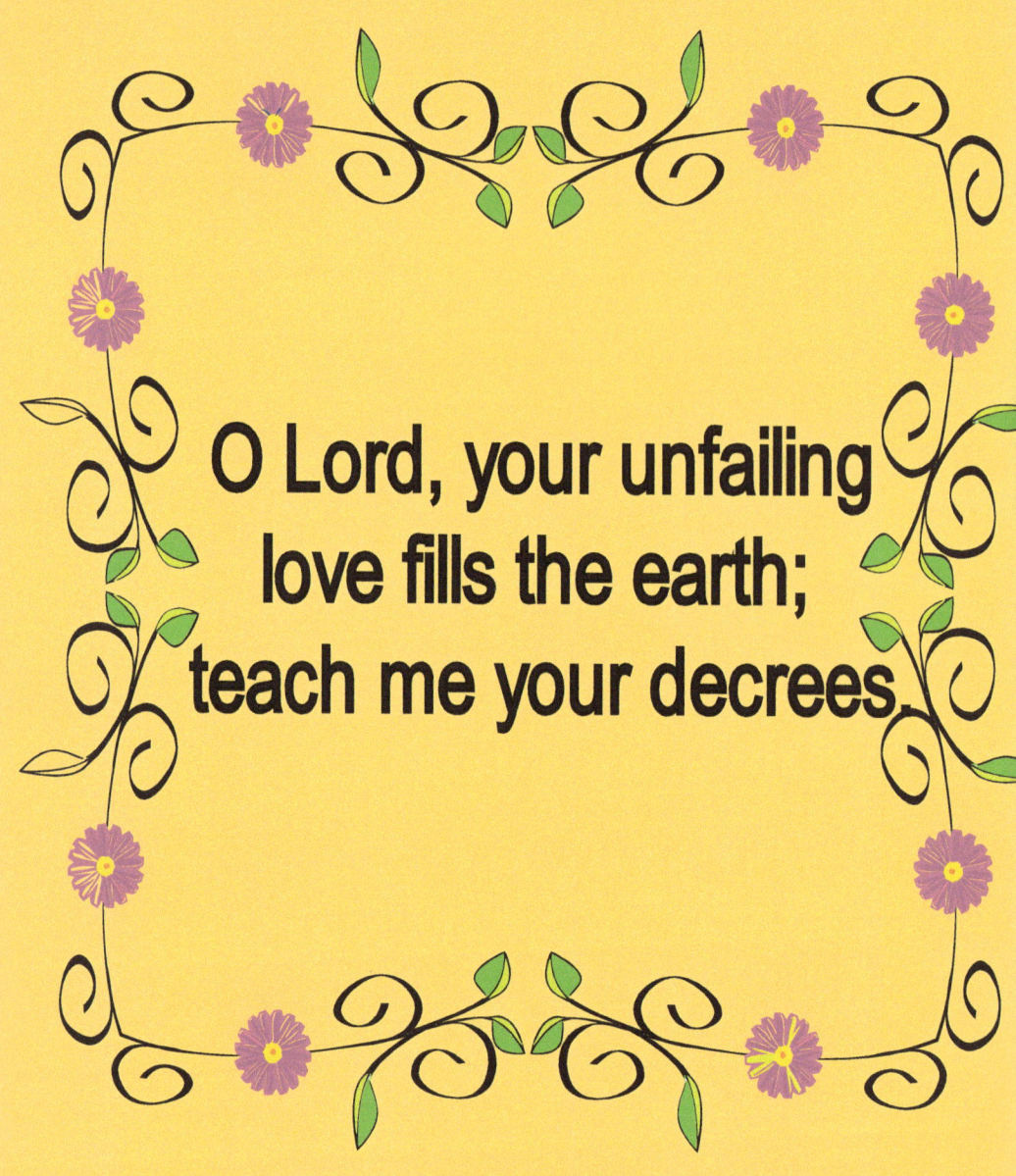

O Lord, your unfailing love fills the earth; teach me your decrees.

Psalm 119:64

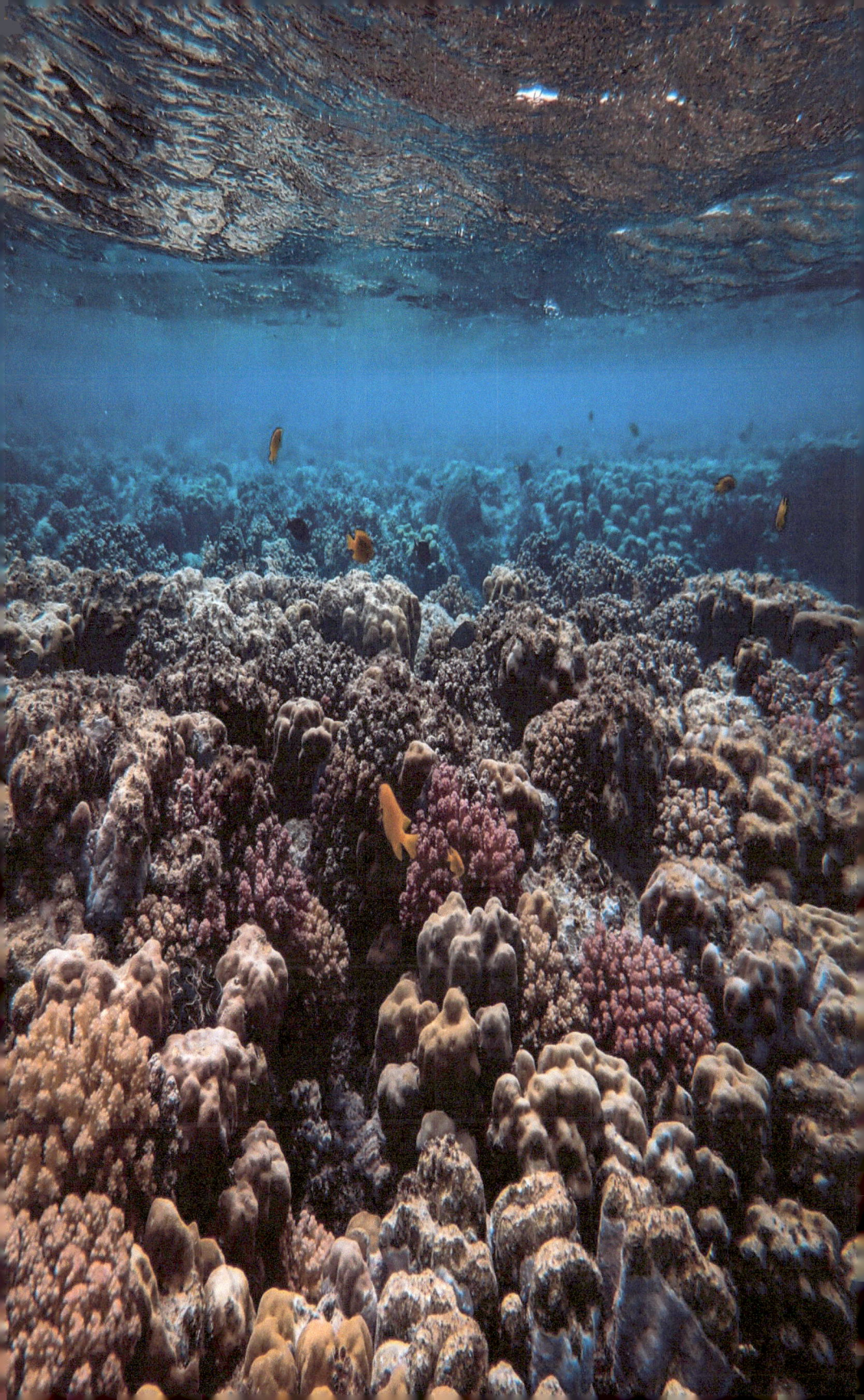

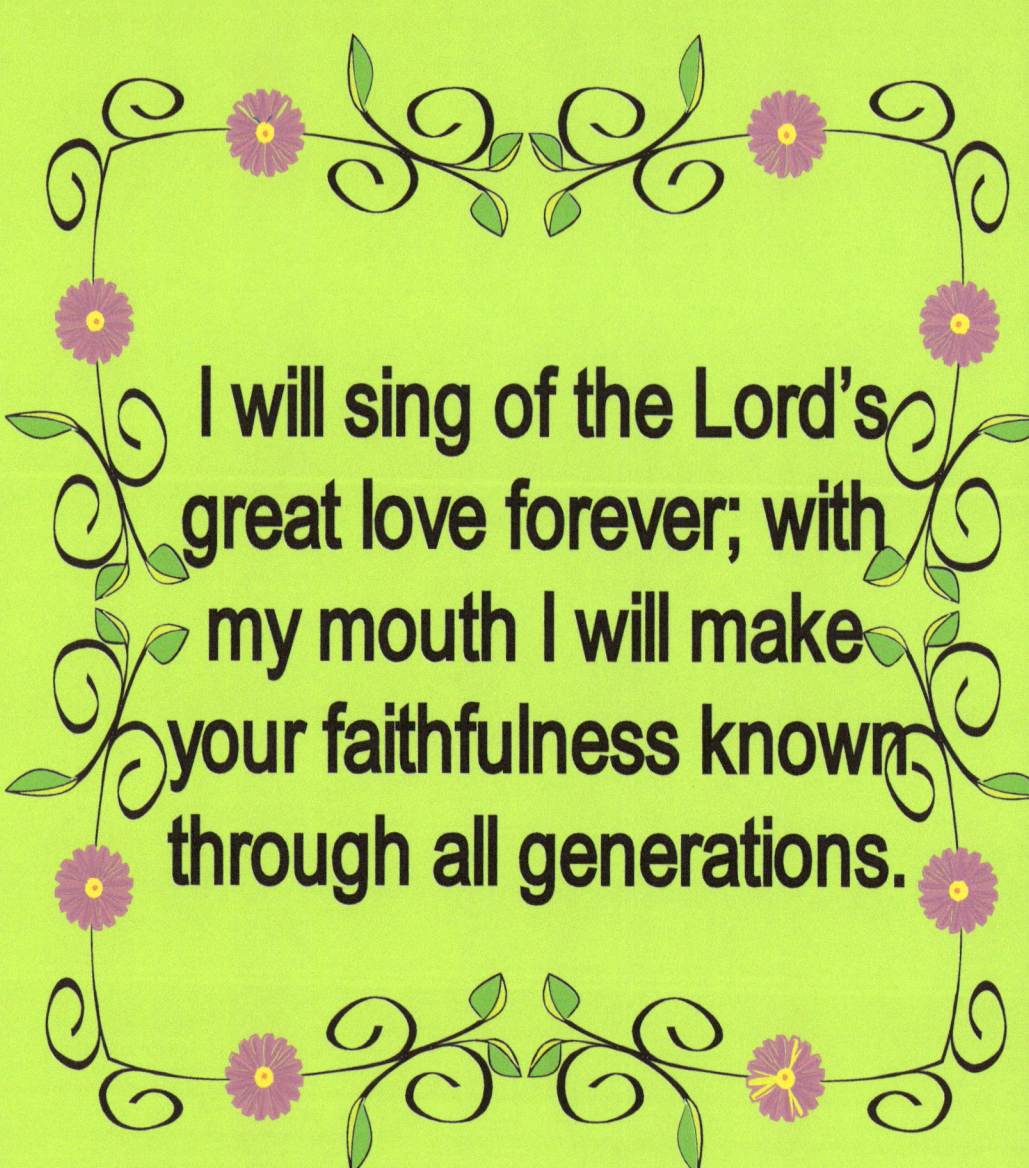

I will sing of the Lord's great love forever; with my mouth I will make your faithfulness known through all generations.

Psalm 89:1

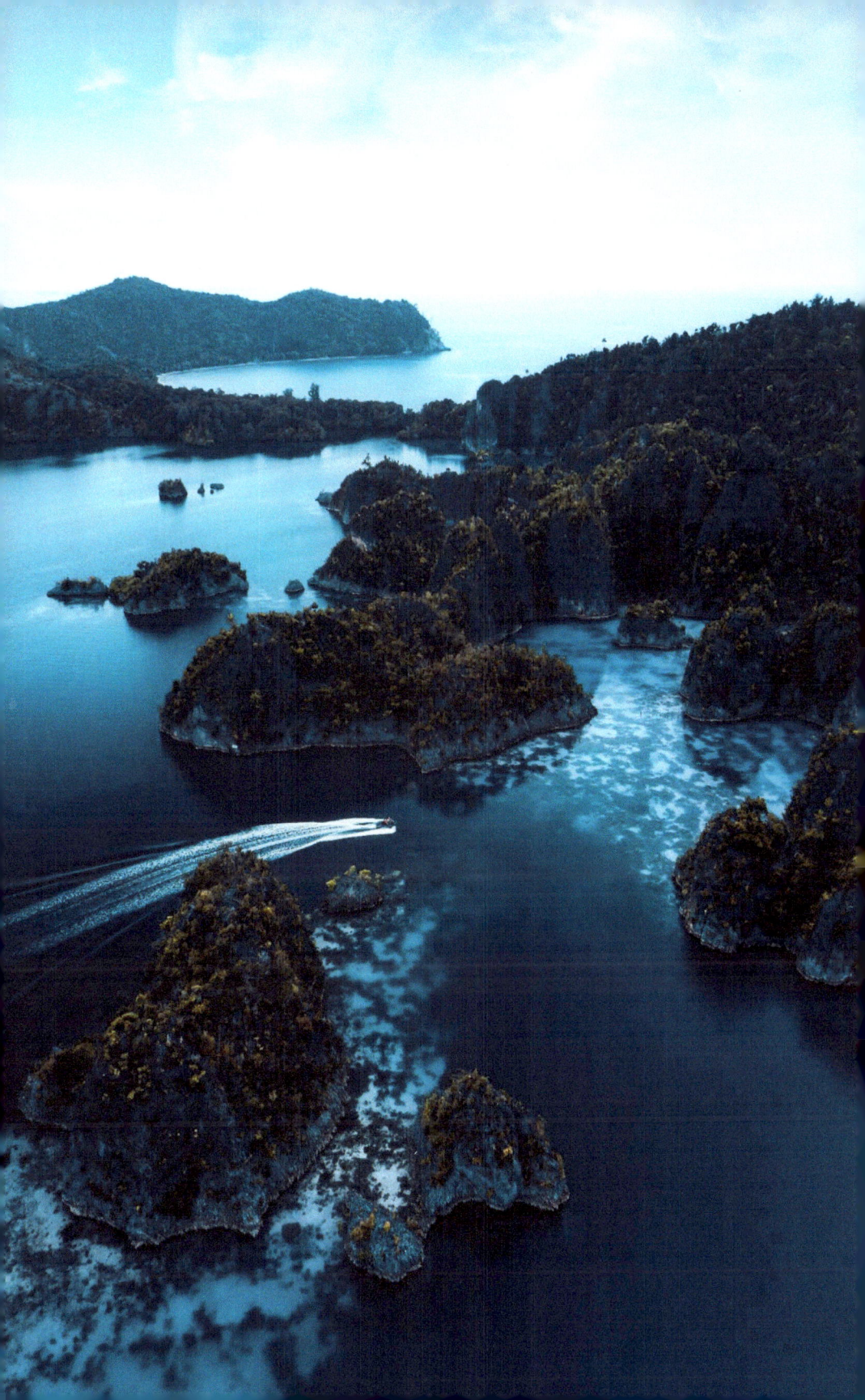

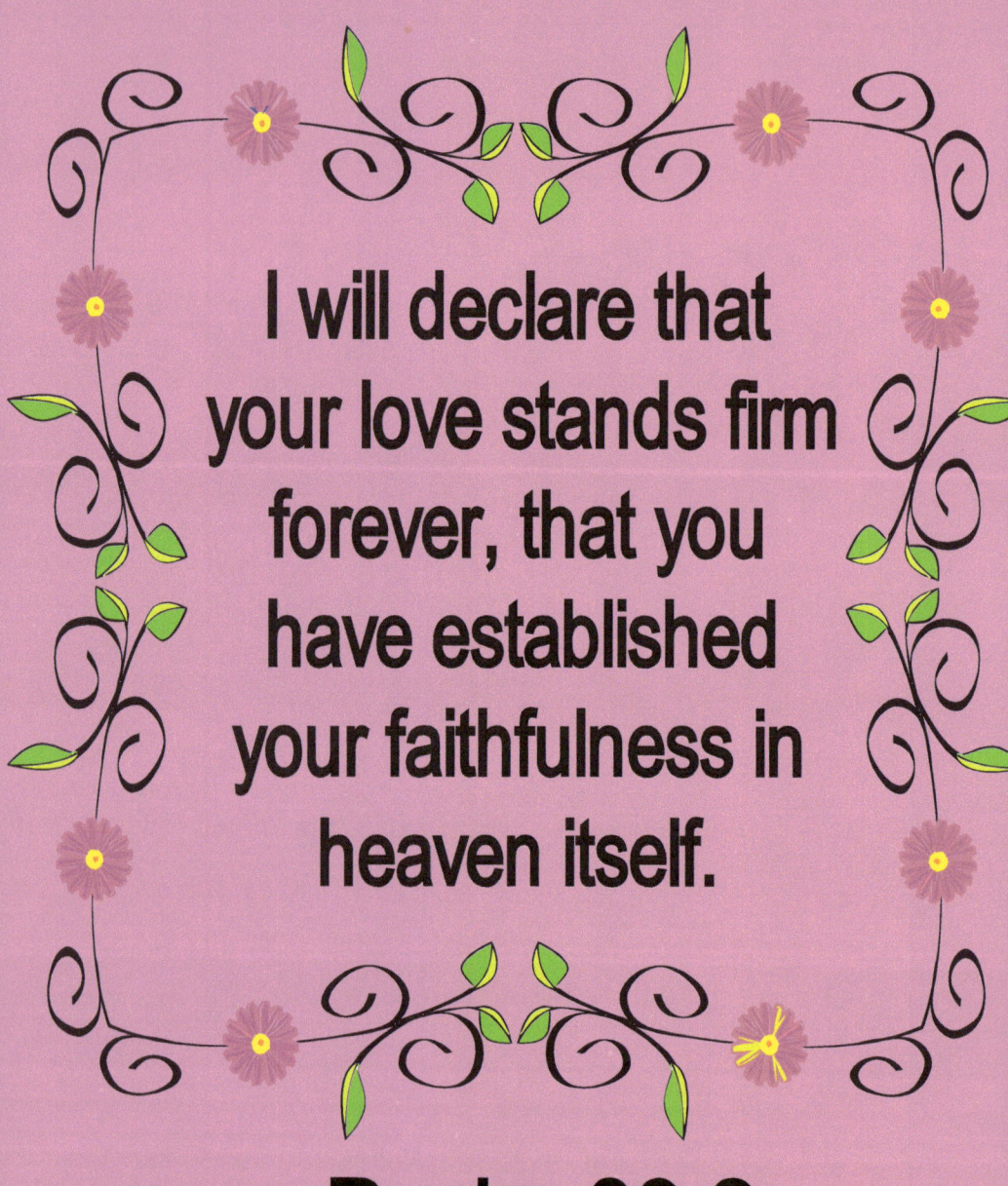

I will declare that your love stands firm forever, that you have established your faithfulness in heaven itself.

Psalm 89:2

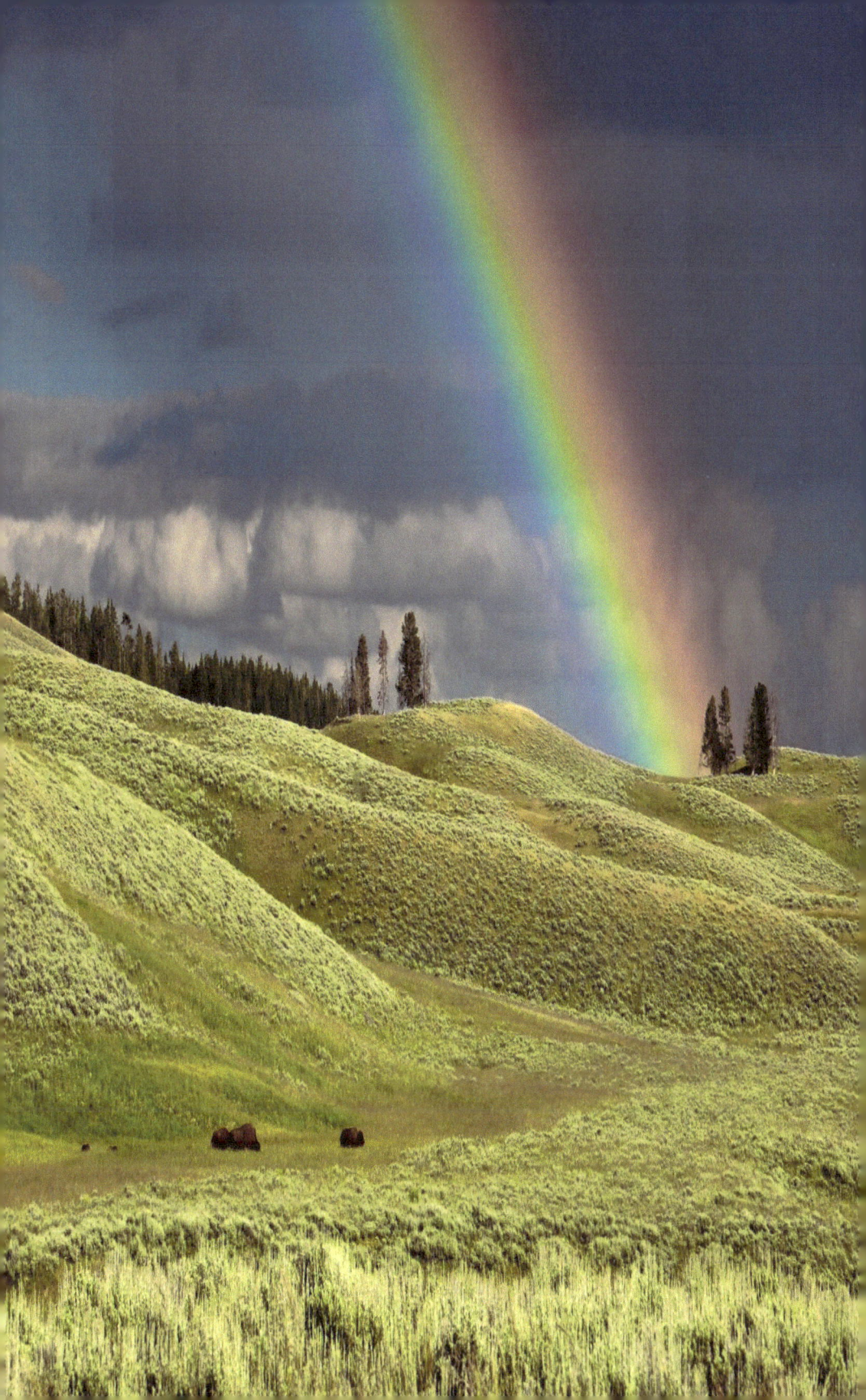

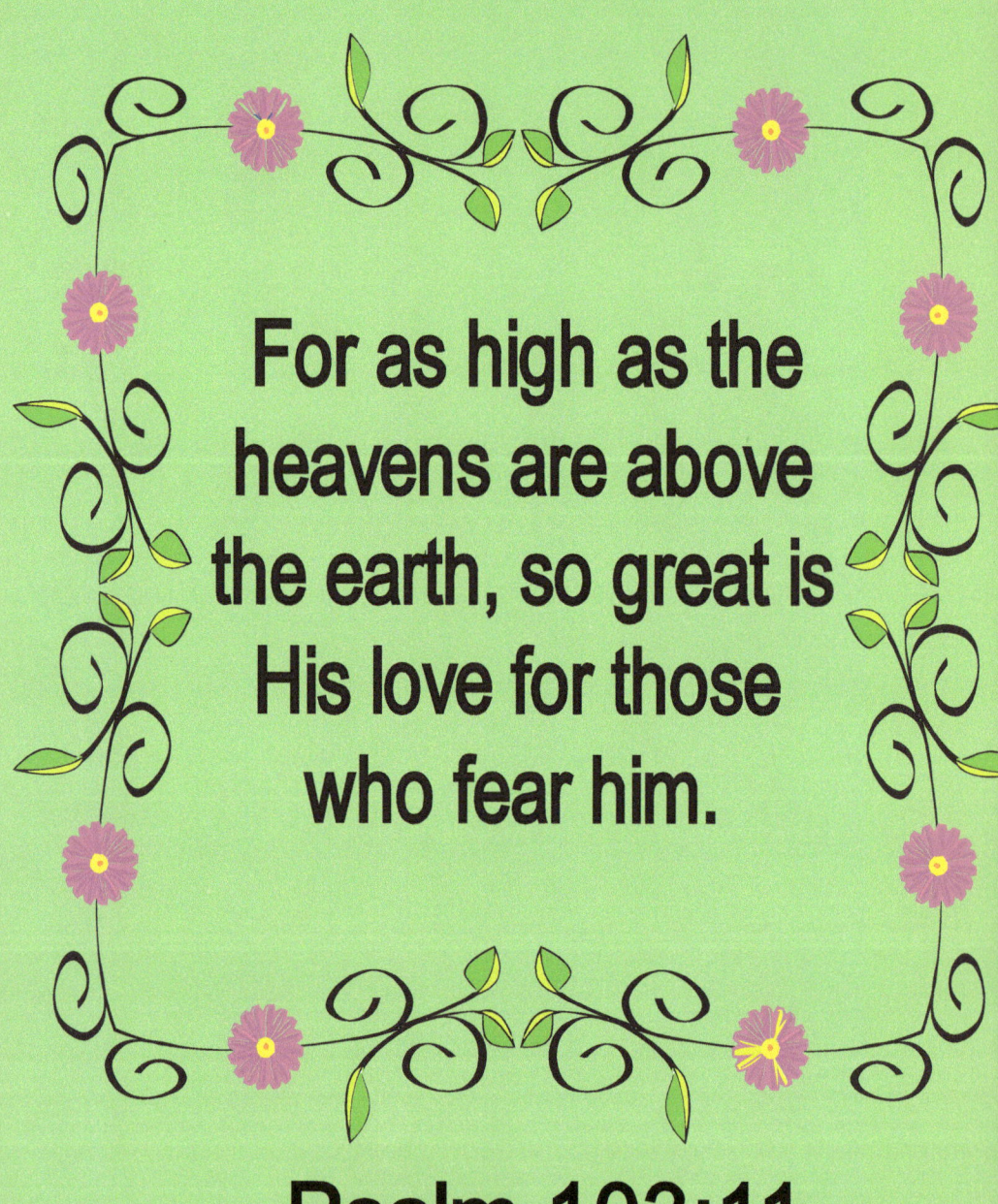

For as high as the heavens are above the earth, so great is His love for those who fear him.

Psalm 103:11

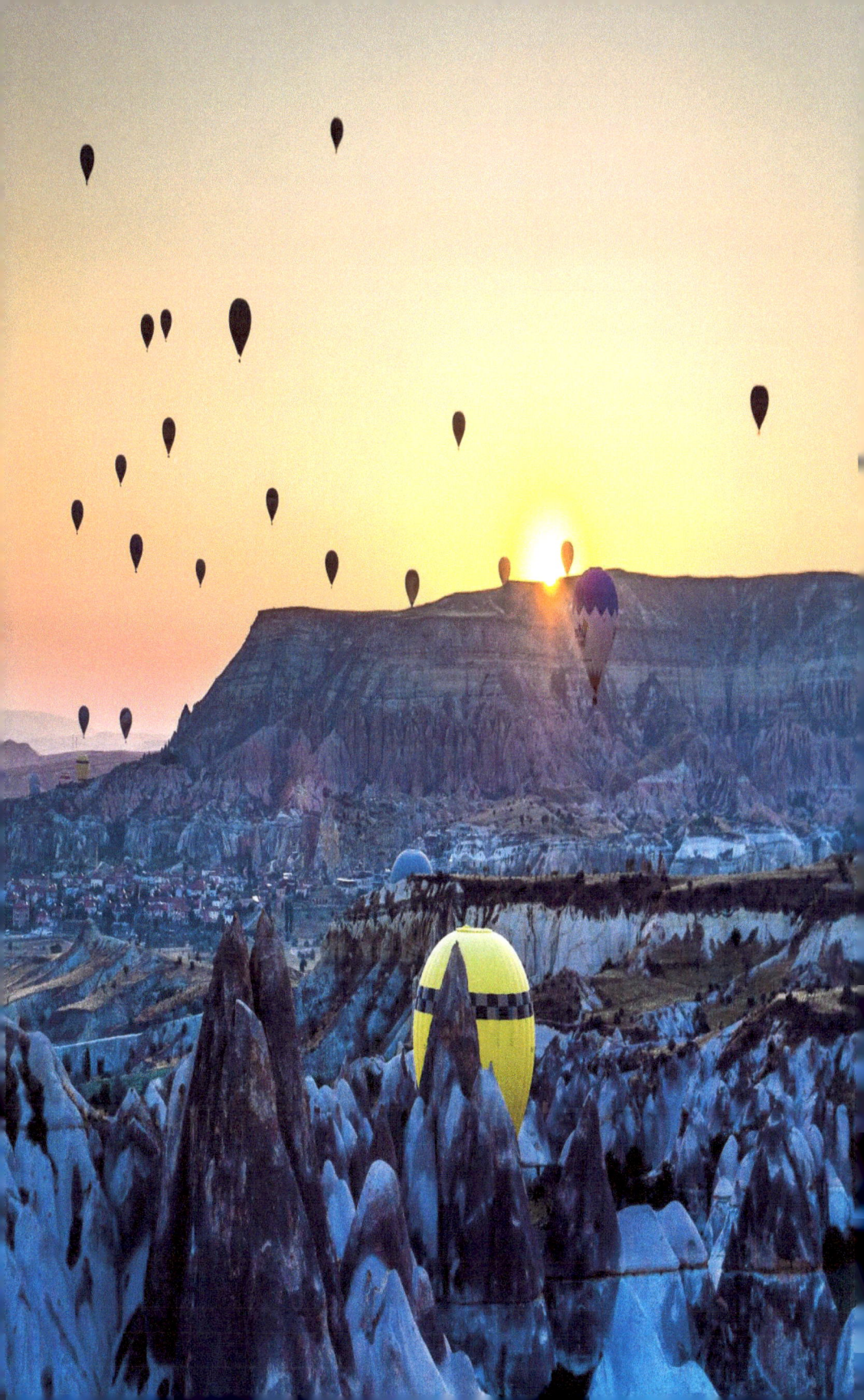

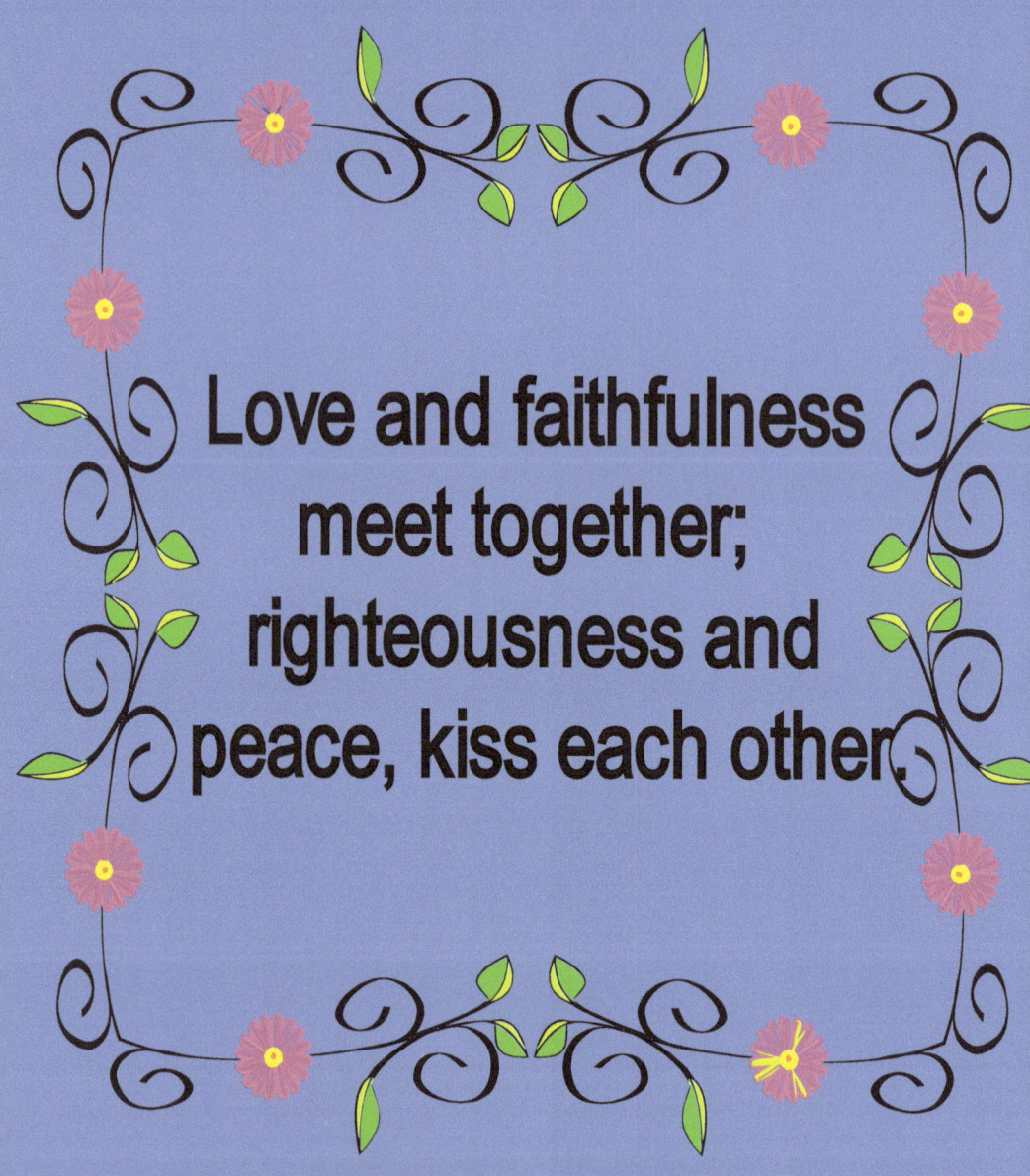

Love and faithfulness meet together; righteousness and peace, kiss each other.

Psalm 85:10

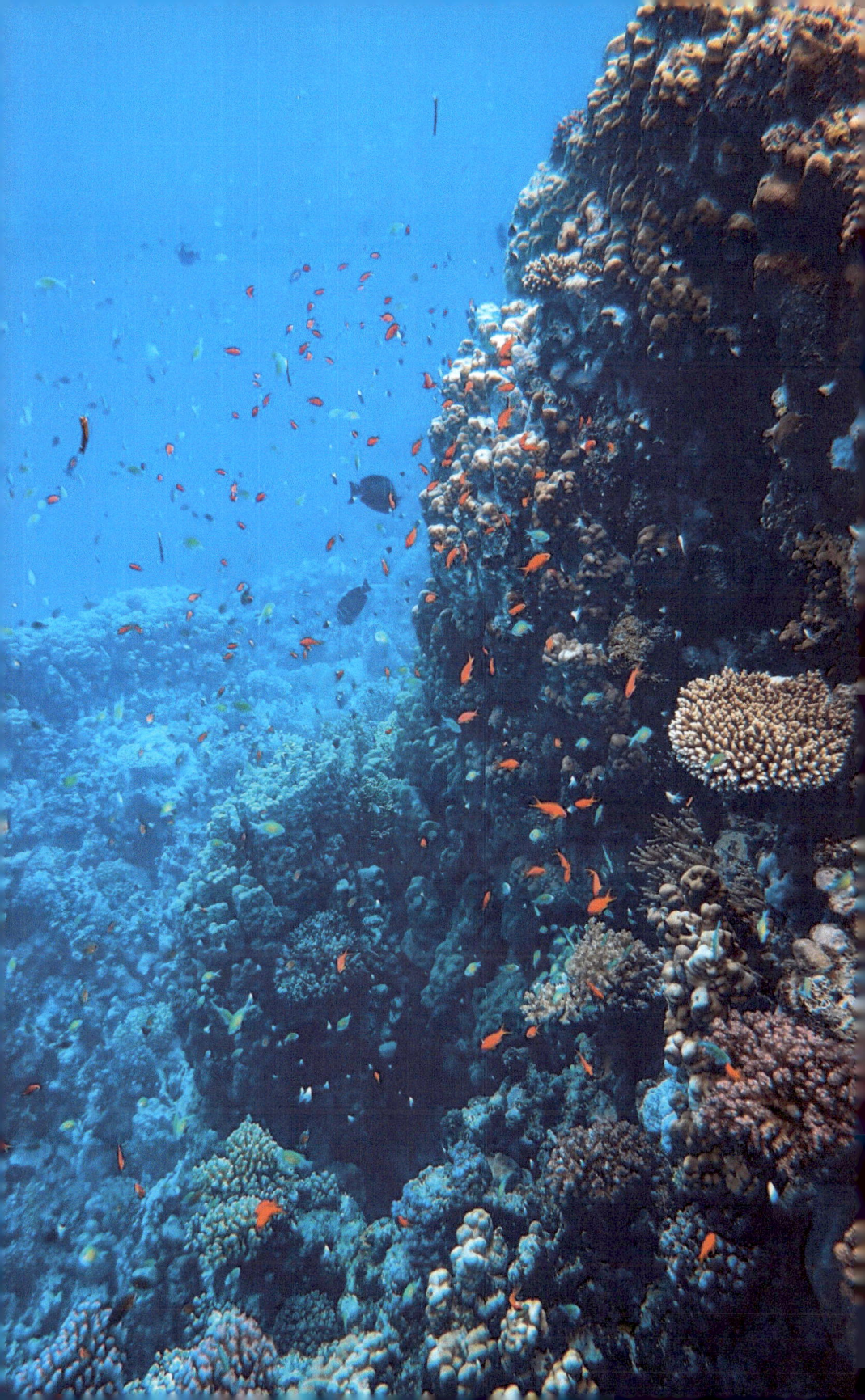

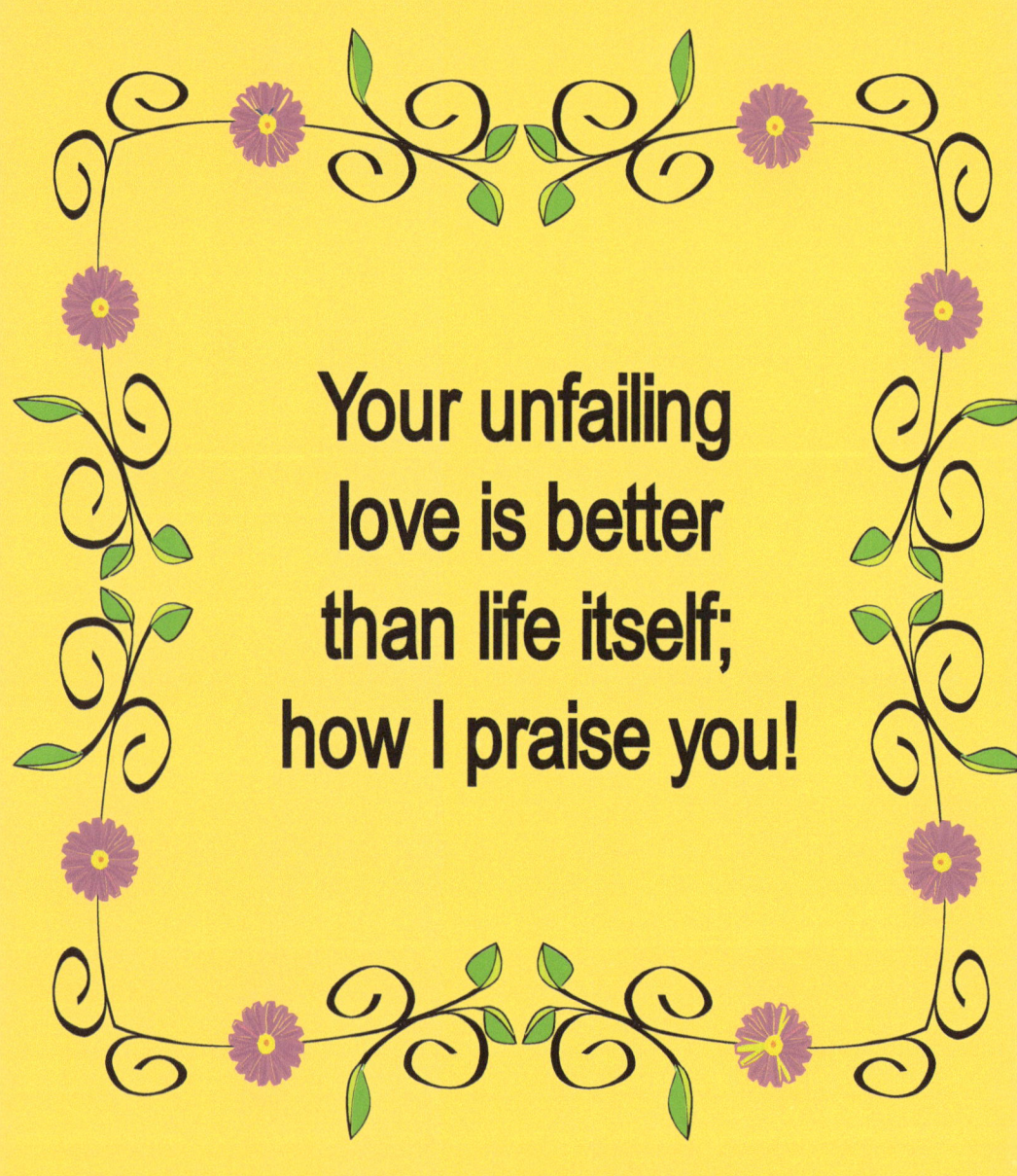

Your unfailing love is better than life itself; how I praise you!

Psalm 63:3

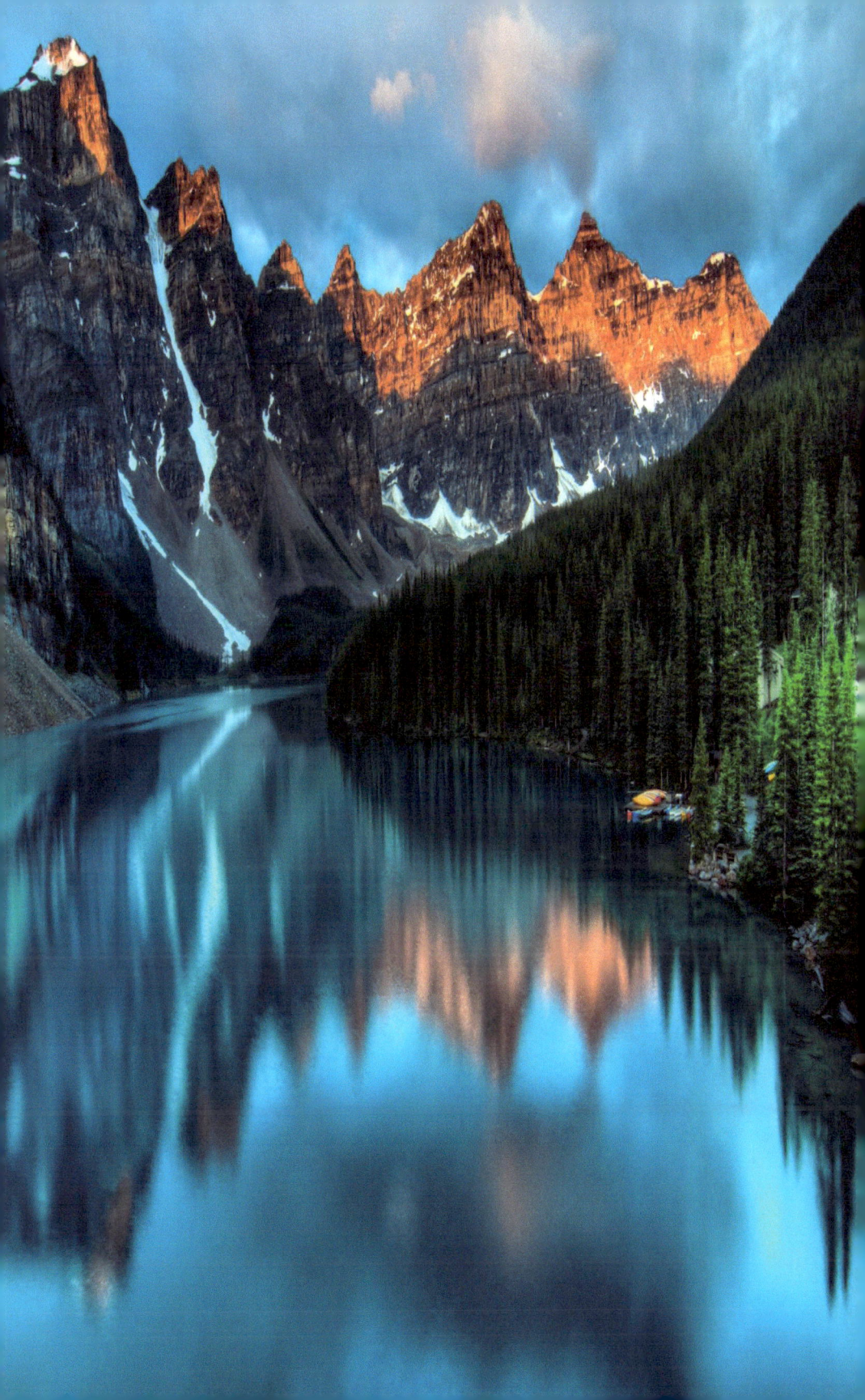

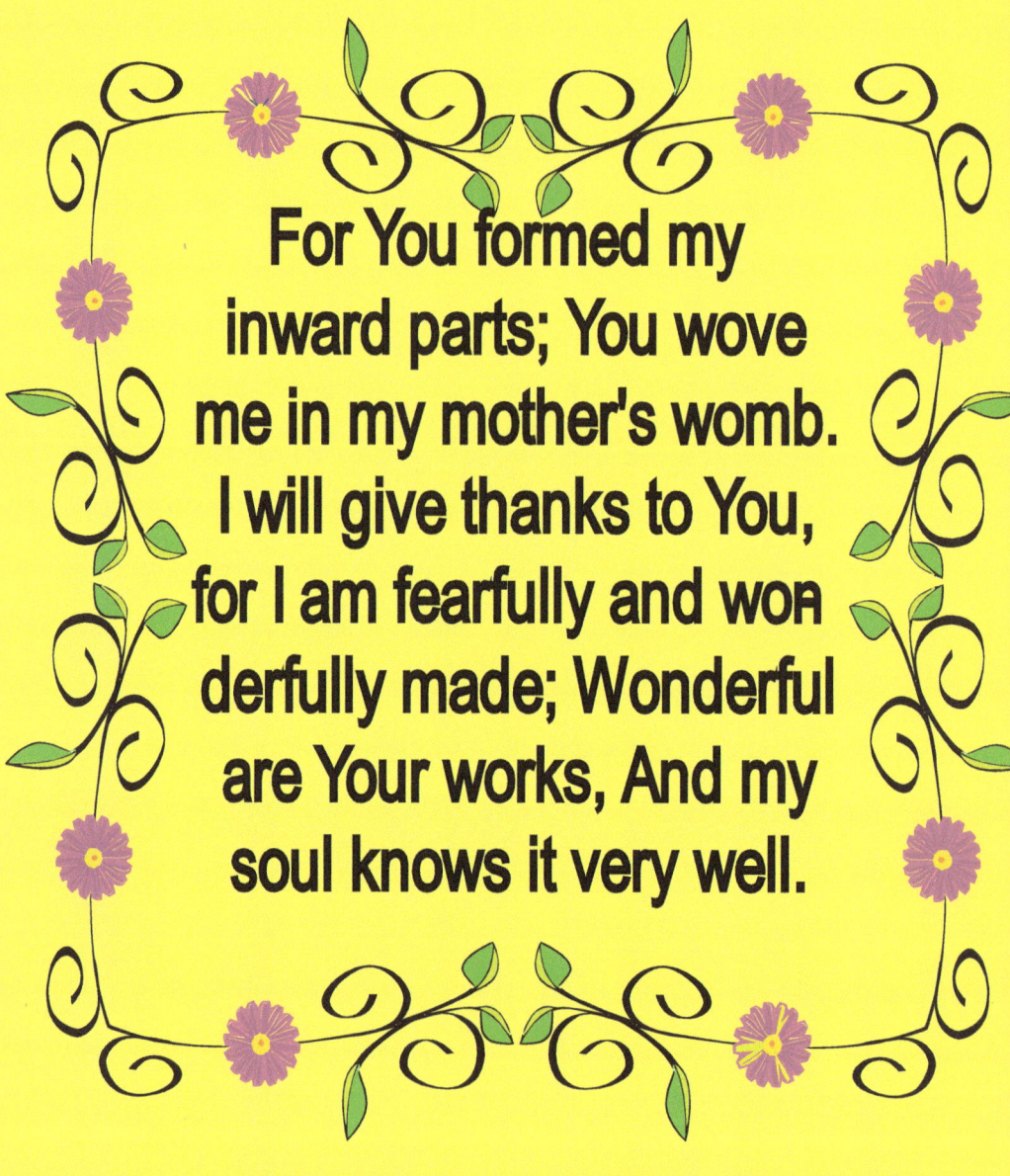

For You formed my inward parts; You wove me in my mother's womb. I will give thanks to You, for I am fearfully and wonderfully made; Wonderful are Your works, And my soul knows it very well.

Psalm 139:13-14

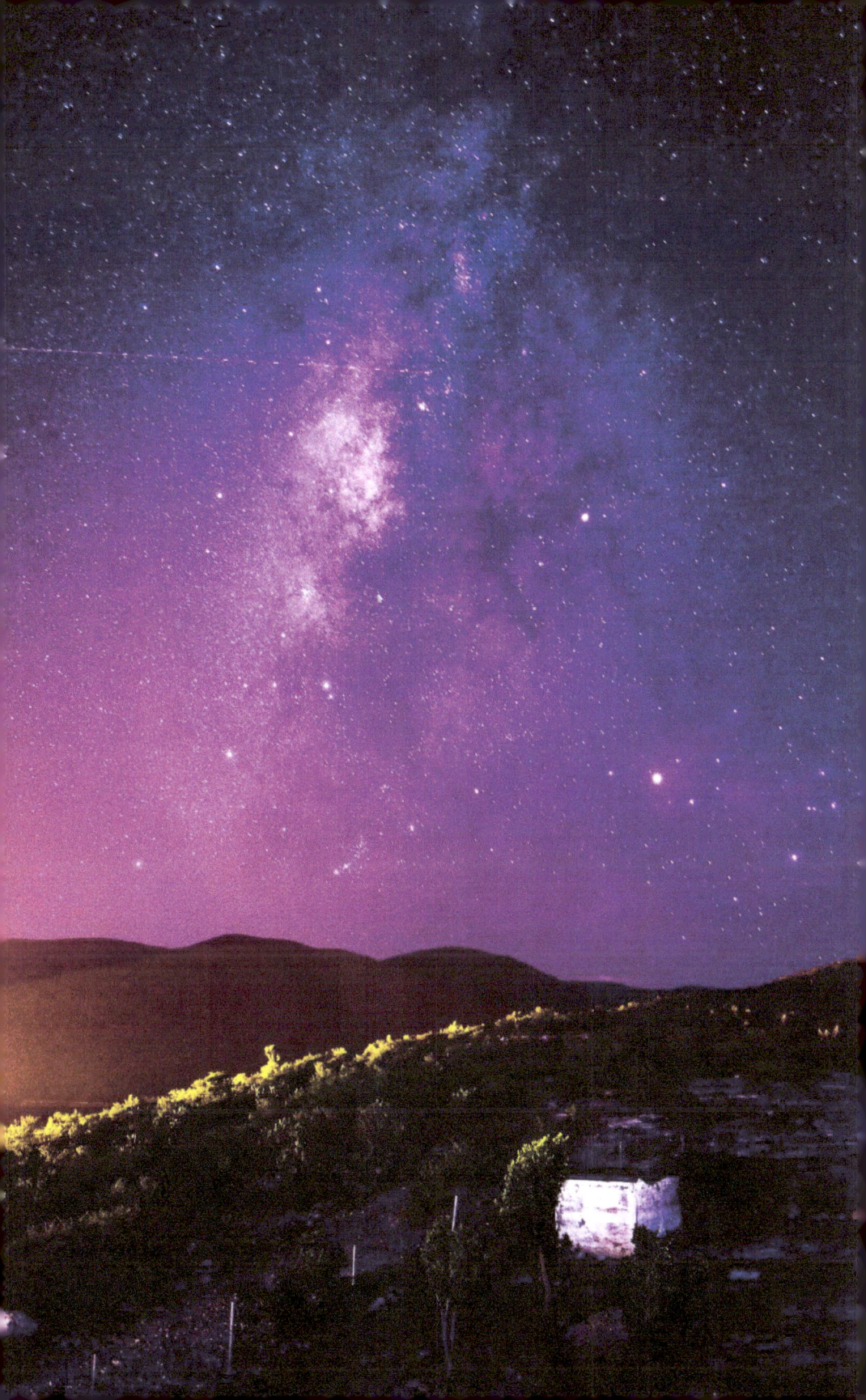

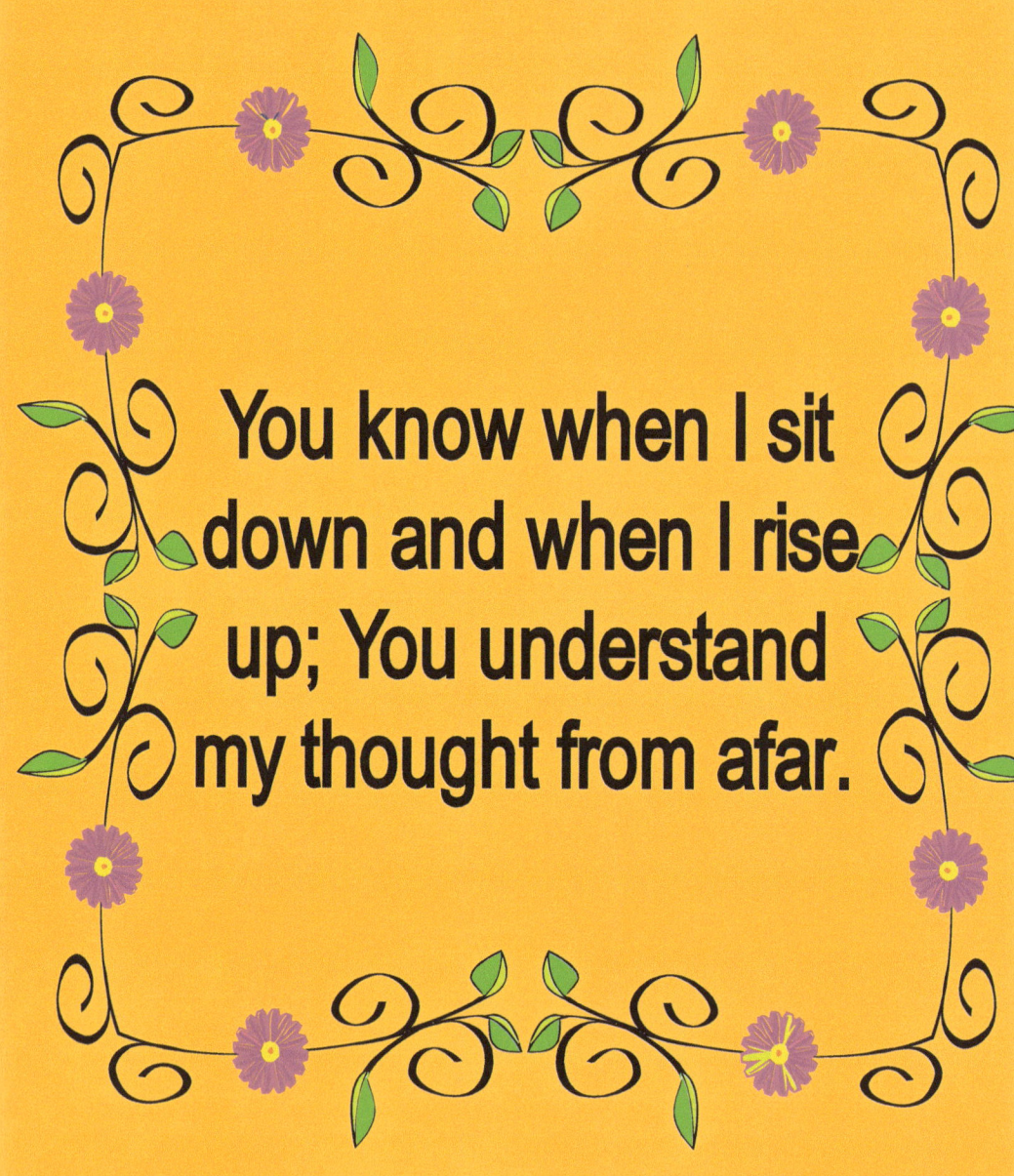

You know when I sit down and when I rise up; You understand my thought from afar.

Psalm 139:2

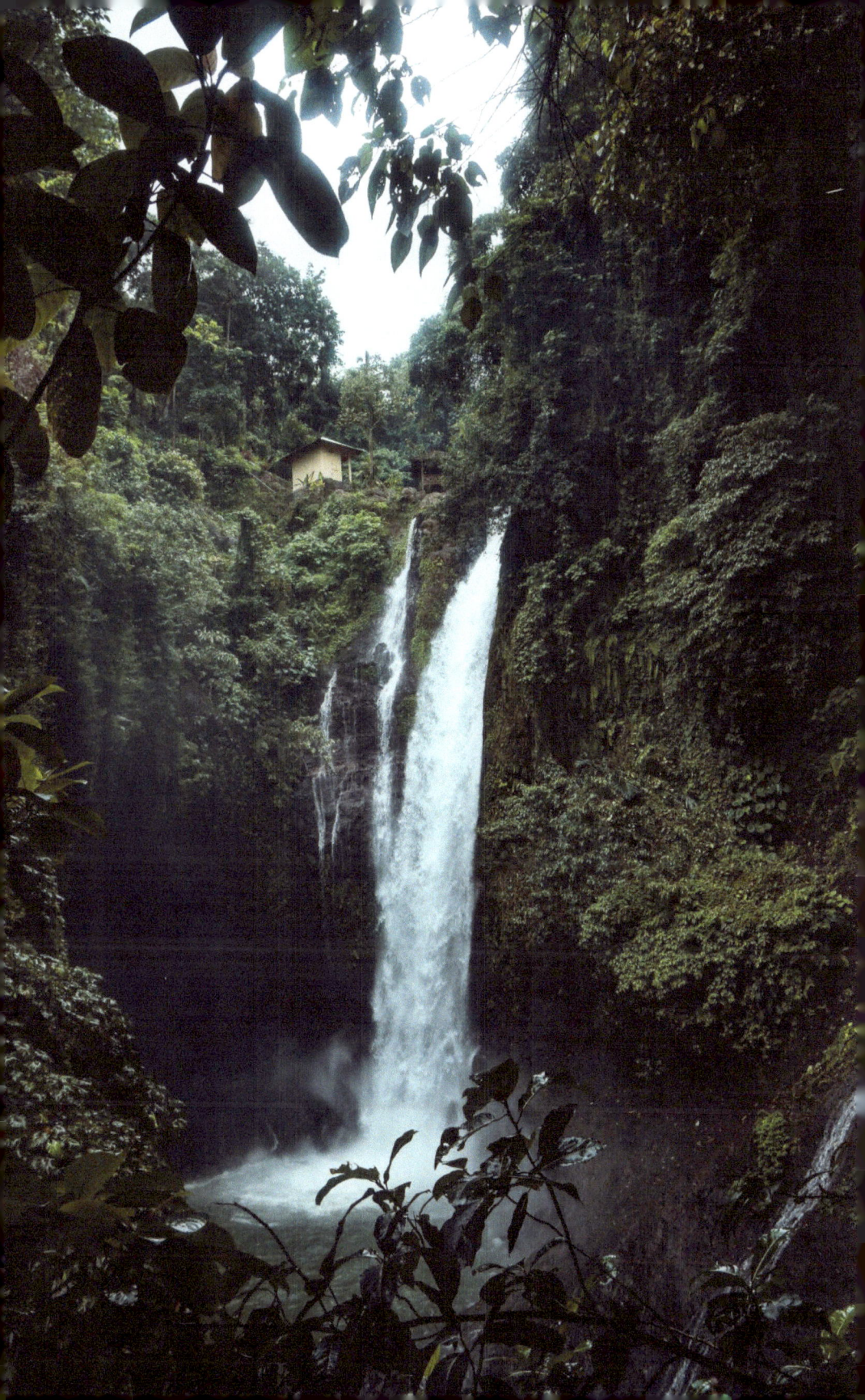

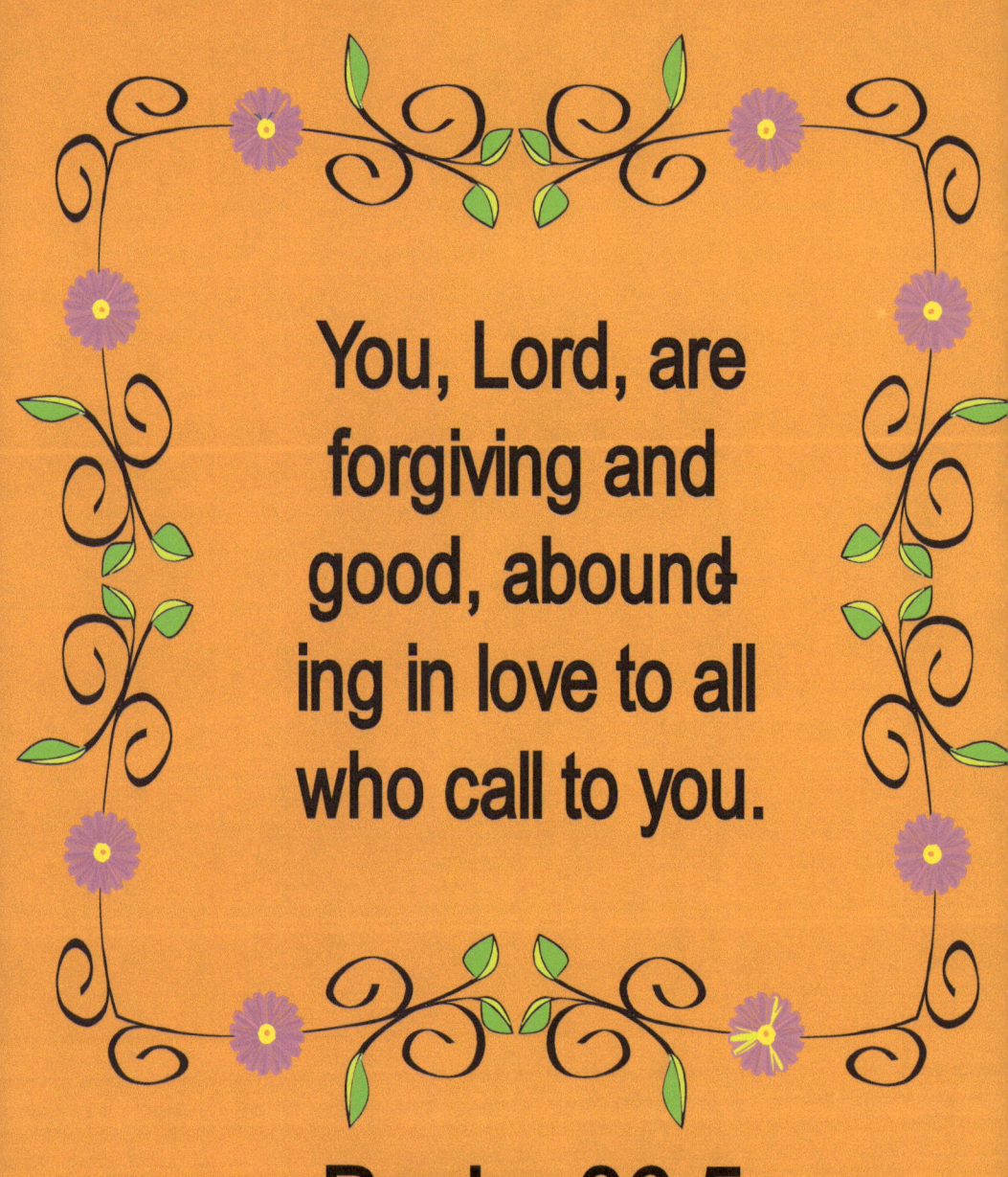

You, Lord, are forgiving and good, abounding in love to all who call to you.

Psalm 86:5

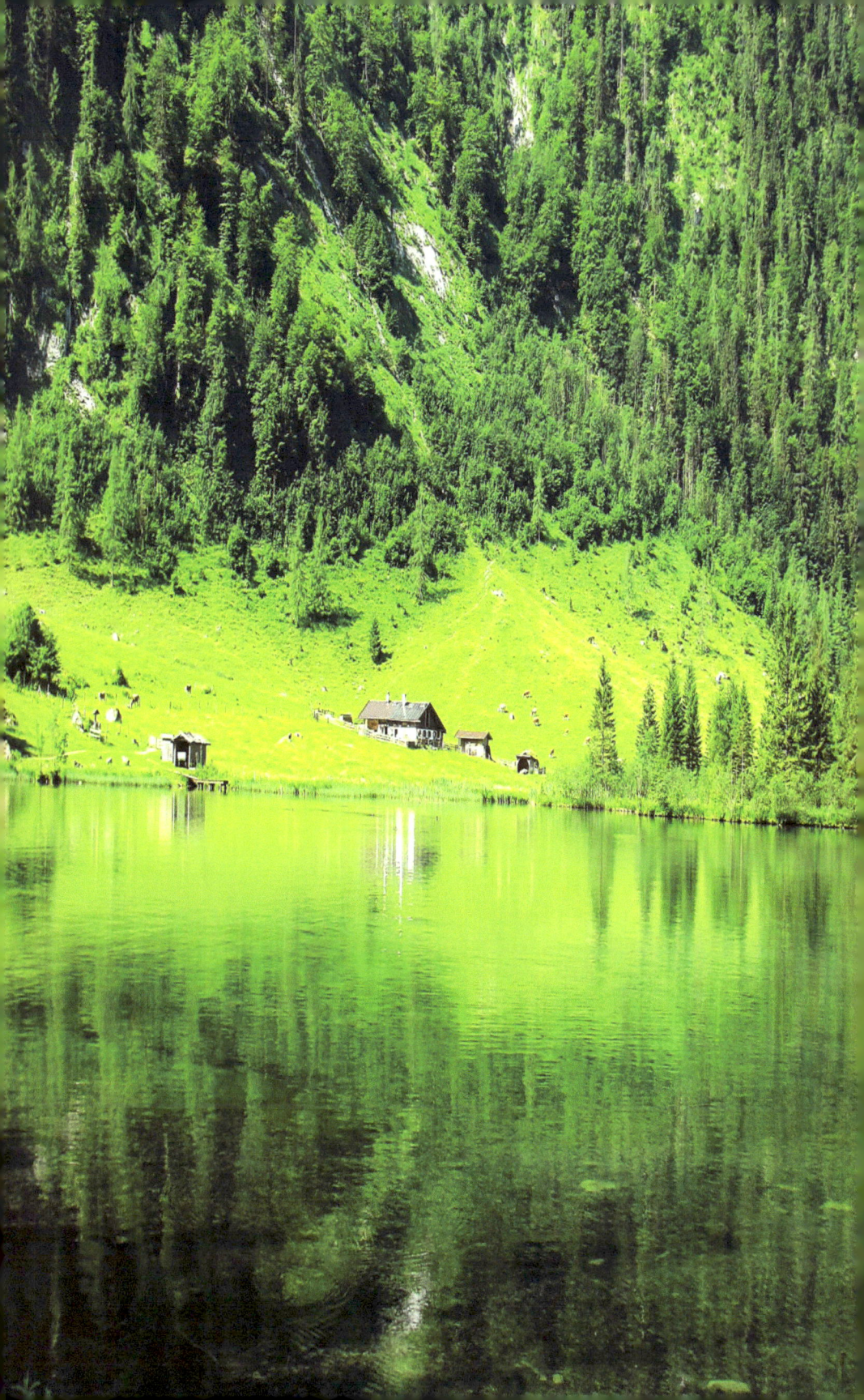

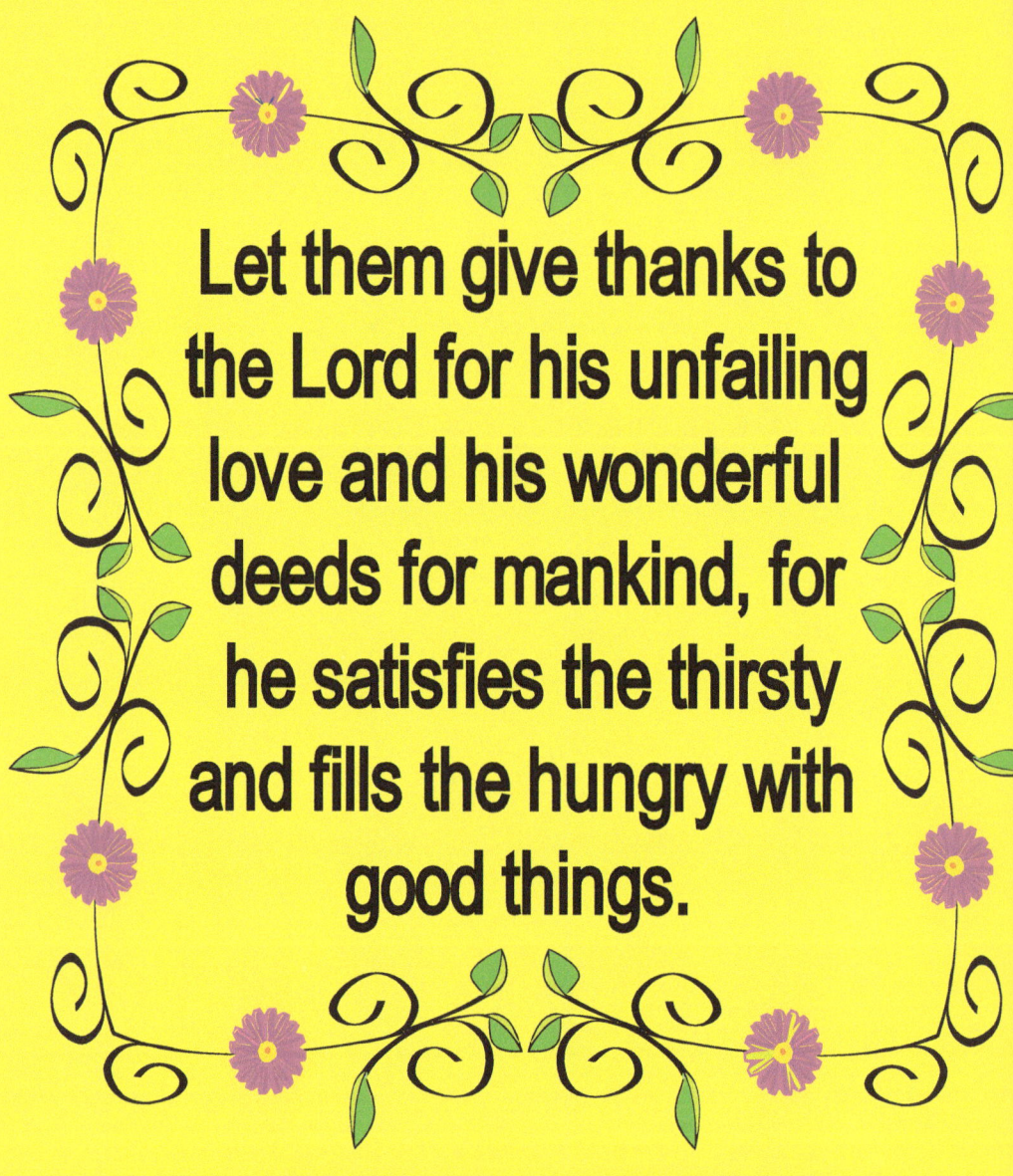

Let them give thanks to the Lord for his unfailing love and his wonderful deeds for mankind, for he satisfies the thirsty and fills the hungry with good things.

Psalm 107:8-9

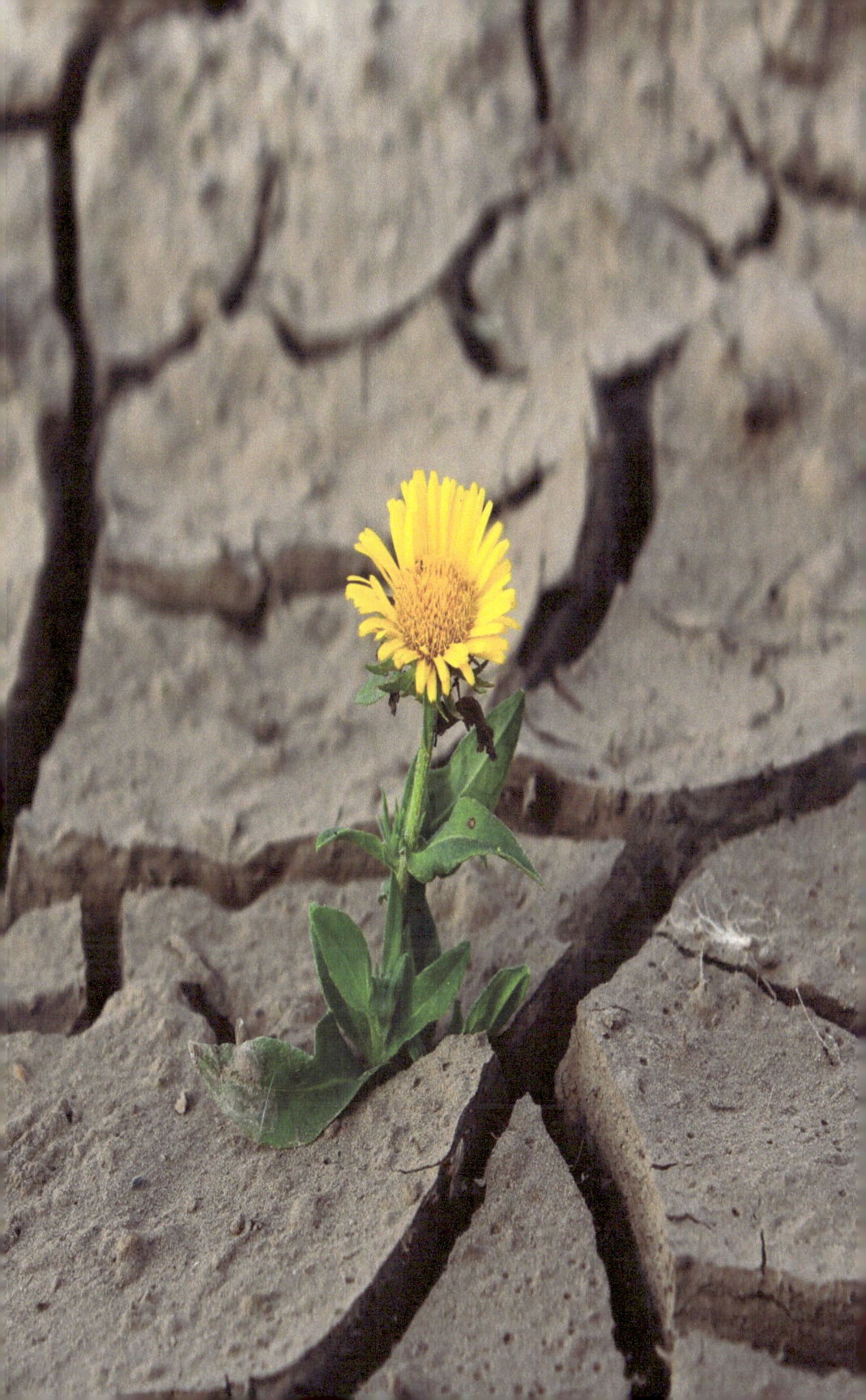

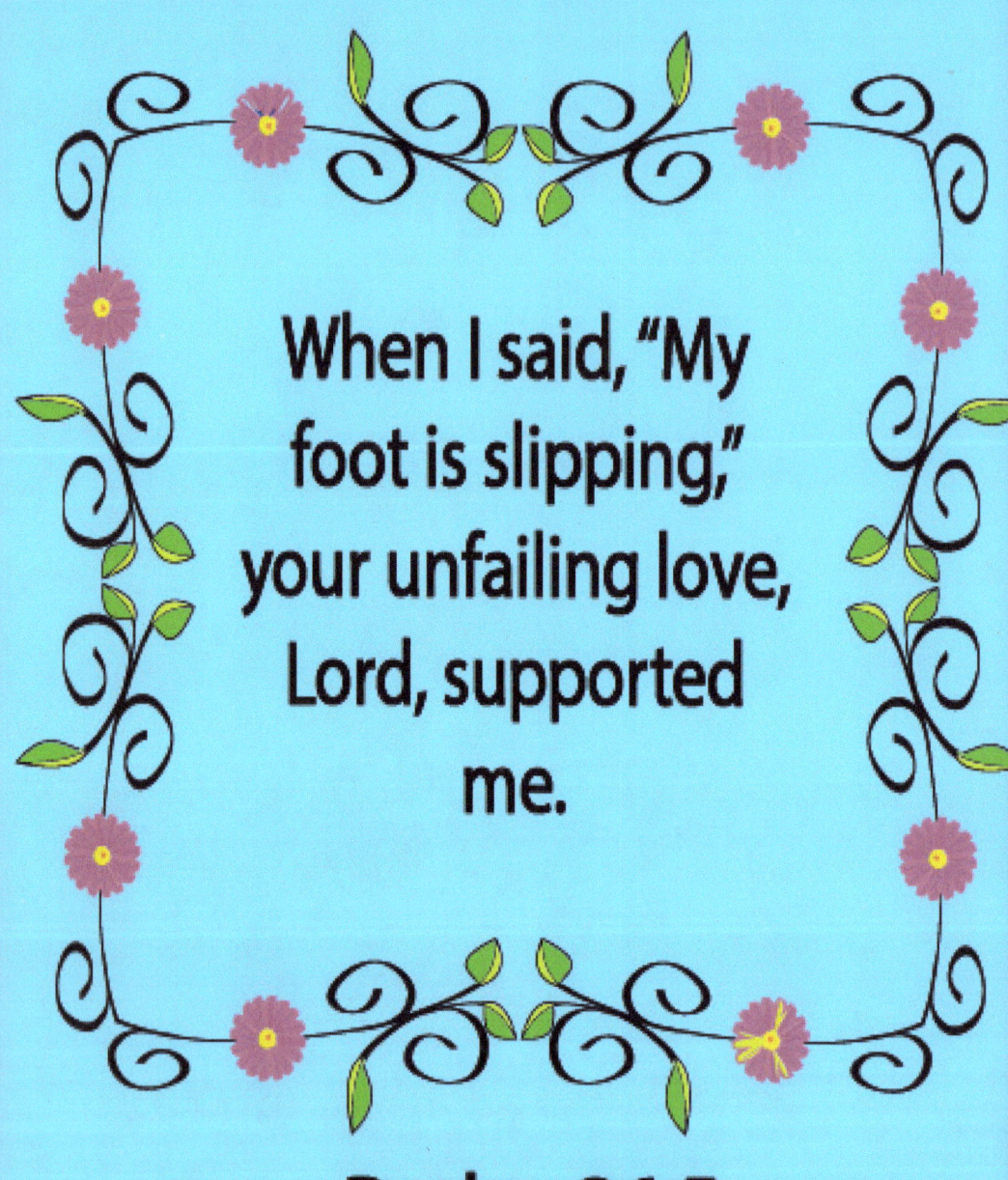

When I said, "My foot is slipping," your unfailing love, Lord, supported me.

Psalm 86:5

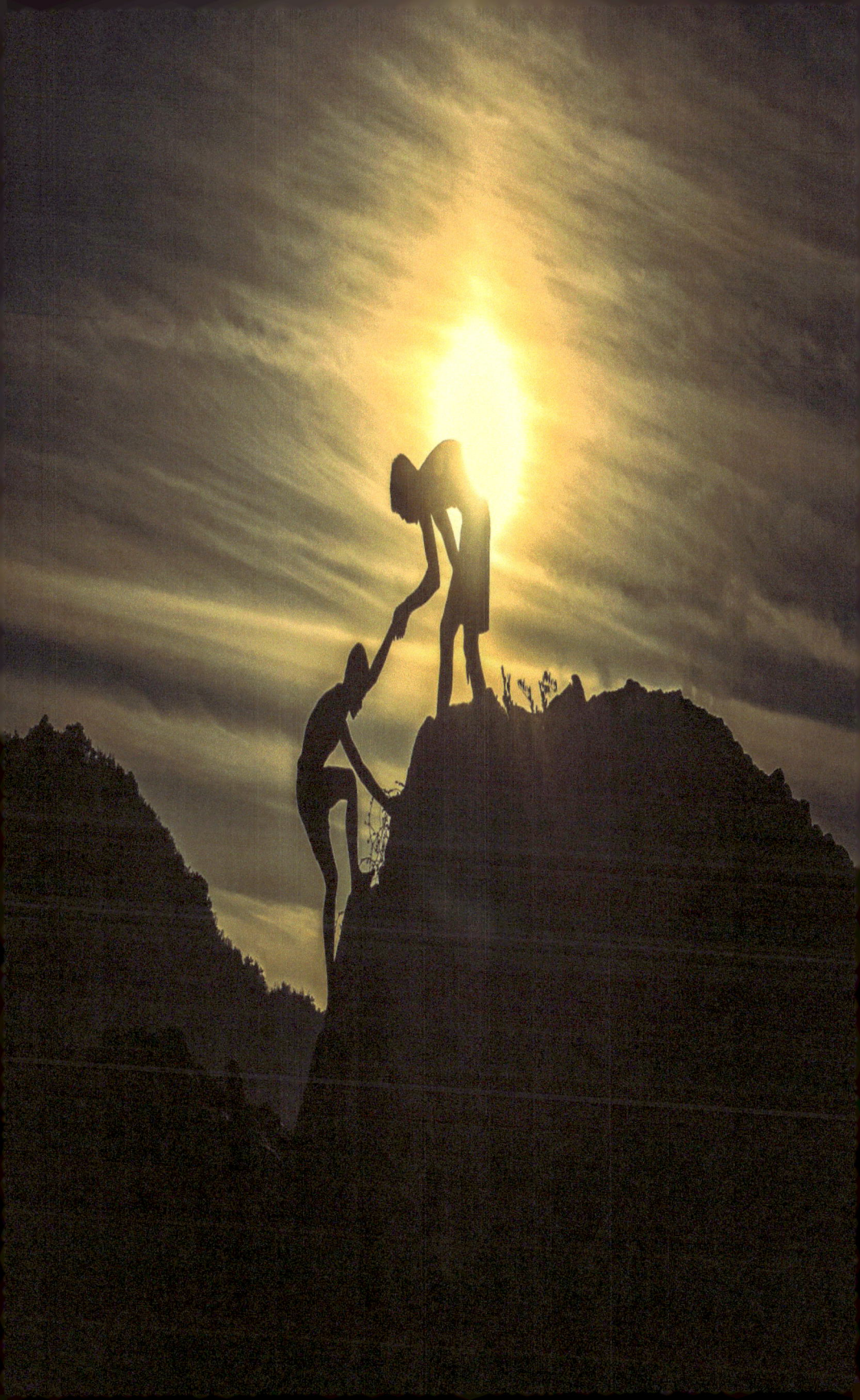

www.ingramcontent.com/pod-product-compliance
Lightning Source LLC
Chambersburg PA
CBHW040252220526
45473CB00001B/457